SEX HABITS

A VITAL FACTOR IN WELL-BEING

DRS. A. BUSCHKE AND F. JACOBSOHN

Dr. Abraham Buschke, specialist in urology and dermatology, was Professor Extraordinary at the University of Berlin for more than twenty years; and was also Director of the Dermatological Section of the Rudolf-Virchow Krankenhaus, one of the largest and most important hospitals in Berlin. His writings on sexual hygiene and venereal disease have been widely published.

Dr. Friedrich Jacobsohn was Dr. Buschke's colleague at the Rudolf-Virchow Krankenhaus, himself specializing in urology. His earlier writing in collaboration with Dr. Buschke was on the subject of venereal disease. Both physicians are greatly impressed and preoccupied with the importance of healthful sex living, as will be readily apparent to readers of the present volume.

DR. G. L. MOENCH

Dr. Gerard L. Moench, who has contributed the foreword to the American edition, is Associate Professor of Gynecology, Associate Attending Gynecologist, and Associate in Pathology at the New York Post Graduate Hospital of Columbia University. He is a Fellow of the American College of Surgeons, a Fellow of the New York Academy of Medicine, and former President of its Section on Gynecology and Obstetrics; a Fellow of the New York Obstetrical Society, etc. He has written extensively on medical subjects, especially on gynecological pathology, and even more particularly on sterility. His work in the latter field has made him known internationally.

SEX HABITS

A VITAL FACTOR IN WELL-BEING

By

A. BUSCHKE, M.D. *and*
F. JACOBSOHN, M.D.

Translated from the German by

EDEN AND CEDAR PAUL

Foreword by

GERARD L. MOENCH, M.D.
New York Post Graduate Hospital
(Columbia University)

NEW YORK
EMERSON BOOKS, INC.

MANUFACTURED IN THE UNITED STATES OF AMERICA

The courts of our country have gone on record as sanctioning rational sex education. They did so in the Stopes case, as well as in the Dennett, during the course of which Federal Judge Augustus N. Hand asserted:

> *". . . The old theory that information about sex matters should be left to chance has greatly changed . . . It may reasonably be thought that accurate information, rather than mystery and curiosity, is better in the long run and is less likely to occasion lascivious thoughts than ignorance and anxiety."*

CONTENTS

CONTENTS

LIST OF ILLUSTRATIONS

FOREWORD TO THE AMERICAN EDITION

THE ancient Greek poets sang of health as the greatest gift of the gods. Today less than ever can we deny the truth of their song, though the idea of what constitutes health has developed into a very much broader concept than it was centuries ago.

Health, which usually we appreciate only when we have it not, is the most important factor in life, not to the individual alone, but to society. Health is, however, not merely a question of organs, normal in the sense that the microscope will reveal no physical aberrations; it means, as well, a proper functioning and interrelation of the various tissues of the body, and their adequate response to physical, chemical, mental and emotional stimuli. That such a definition of health includes normal sex functions is, or should be, self evident.

I believe it is not exaggerating to say that disturbances of the sexual apparatus cause more mental anguish and emotional upsets, aside from physical suffering, than any other lesions. And yet, until recently, the forces of taboo, intolerance and hypocrisy have succeeded in banishing instruction in this most important domain of sex, to the realm of chance and gossip, with the result that fancy and superstition have replaced factual knowledge.

It is high time that this state of affairs be remedied. It is high time that the warped individual to whom sex and immorality are synonymous, be restrained from persecuting serious works on sexual problems. Of late there is indeed some hope of finally accomplishing this, for it certainly is a sign of progress that a jury conviction of Mary Ware Dennett, for selling her pamphlet "The Sex Side of Life," was overturned by the judges of the Circuit Court of Appeals. The sagacious decision handed down by Federal Judge John M. Woolsey in the Stopes case was another step forward. What we need is not a veiling and concealment of sex, but sane and unbiased instruction which, in a simple, and yet in a complete and authoritative manner, will discuss the problems of sex, and emphasize the importance of normal sex functions to the general bodily health.

It is with such a purpose in view that the present volume, now admirably translated into English, was written by two German physicians. The book offers, to my mind, one of the sanest discussions yet presented to the public. One may not agree with all the authors' views. One may wish that the deleterious influence of venereal diseases on the individual and on the offspring were stressed more. One may even consider that the discussion of the "double standard" is rather futile (because the essentially monogamous psyche of the average woman is, after all, not a product of fetters or freedom), though admittedly there is much food for consideration in the carefully measured views of the authors. These, however, are but minor points in a generally excellent volume. The anatomical chapters alone would amply justify its publication. Of course there may be some who will object to illustrations of the sex organs, in a volume for lay consumption, on grounds of immorality. Let us gently remind such objectors that, after all, the immorality resides not in the really magnificent plates, but in their own minds.

Aside from the strictly anatomical and physiological chapters of the book, the chapter on puberty is worth learning by heart by all parents, and the discussions on the sex impulse in man and woman will give increased understanding to those contemplating marriage. That a chapter of the volume has been devoted to sex abnormalities, I consider most fortunate. There is no field where ignorance is more prevalent than here, so that sex abnormalities have become the subject of coarse jokes, or oftentimes are indiscriminately classed as crimes.

Some of the authors' remarks on the misinterpretation of the work of Freud have struck a responsive chord in my heart. Maltreated and mutilated, the theories of Freud have been bandied about by the untrained—even in best sellers—for untrained, and often half-baked readers; until the work of a really brilliant man has, for many, come to be synonymous with filth.

It is tempting to add further discussion, but the book speaks for itself. The rabid sex reformers will be disappointed, some purists will perhaps be shocked, but to the balanced reader this sane and unbiased discussion of sex, its functions and problems, will assuredly be welcome.

GERARD L. MOENCH, M.D.

New York City
August, 1933

CHAPTER I

Introductory

Sexology, the science of the sexual life and activities of living beings, is not a sharply limited department of human knowledge, for it shades at the edges into the domains of philosophy, biology, medicine, law, political economy, and statistics. The theologian, the educationist, and the judge all need a knowledge of it in their daily work. Day by day, however, we encounter tragical examples of their ignorance in such matters. The present work, therefore, is designed, not merely to diffuse precise knowledge about the life of sex, but also to aid in preventing the mischief that so often results from injustice in the law courts where sexual matters are concerned. The authors hope to assist in reducing the extent to which natural impulses and activities are wrongly condemned. With no less emphasis, however, shall we inveigh against uncontrol and levity in sexual concerns—against the licence which many claim as the right of the younger generation.

In contrast with the views which prevailed twenty years ago, it is now frequently held that women no less than men are entitled " to gratify their impulses freely ". It used to be regarded as self-evident that the right to pre-conjugal sexual activities, and also to sexual relations of a fugitive and transient nature, must be exclusively reserved for men. What was called the " double standard " of morality then prevailed. That which was allowed to a young man was forbidden to a young woman. There were, indeed, attempts to challenge this double standard, and to declare that sexual freedom was no less permissible for women than for men ; but they never gained general support. From the other side came endeavours to induce young men to renounce pre-conjugal sexual activity, the demand for " masculine purity " being voiced by groups of eccentrics, usually consisting of persons holding strict religious views, and eager to win disciples among university students. The majority of young men, however, whether of the upper, the middle, or the working class, gave free rein to their sexual impulses. Gratification was sought in the embraces of prostitutes, avowed or clandestine ; or else, as far as a minority was concerned, in unions which were somewhat more lasting, but were none the less fugitive—in " intimacies ".

During the war of 1914–18 and in the post-war period, the double standard in sexual matters broke down, young women claiming and exercising the same freedom as young men. The view that what was permissible to a man must be permissible to a woman as well, seemed a logical deduction to many of those who were fighting for the equal rights of women in the economic and social fields. There were many additional factors of the changes in theory and practice. The economic upheaval of the last ten or fifteen years (accentuated in Germany, above all, by inflation) brought young men and young women of all classes into closer contact one with another under conditions in which there was far less supervision than of yore. Furthermore, the traditional standards of sexual conduct were undermined in consequence of the recognition that in many other respects the most venerable traditions were outworn. What has been called "an intoxication of uncontrol" spread through all domains of social life; there was no longer any attempt to resist impulse; the search for pleasure became universal. Young men, therefore, no longer had the smallest difficulty in finding sexual partners ready to enter into temporary relationships; with the result that, in the rising generation, it was largely taken as a matter of course that the sexes had an equal right to early indulgence. This change of outlook found expression both in public and in private life. For instance, in the course of a decade there occurred a gradual change in opinion as to what was right and proper for girls and young women in the way of dress, make-up, etc. It must not be supposed that middle-class and working-class women who follow the prevailing fashion in the use of the lipstick are fully aware that they are adopting a means of attraction which was previously left for prostitutes. There were, no doubt, other motives at work besides the instinctive desire to comply with the often perverted taste of their male companions. There was an element of convenience in the bobbing of hair and in the wearing of extremely short skirts. Still, the sexual components in these changes of fashion must not be overlooked. In the long run we think that the obliteration of all conventional standards as to what is seemly in social life will be found to be intolerable. During the period we are now considering, the dance, which essentially is symbolical of sexual self-expression and sexual self-defence and is only incidentally a delight in rhythm, became so manifestly erotic that one did not need to be a prude to be forced into regarding this over-emphasis of the sexual as morbid. Besides, during a period of great economic stress, the devotion of so much time and energy and money to dancing becomes a serious matter. Nor must it be forgotten that private and public dances, which used to be occasions when young people could become acquainted with one another as a step to marriage, are now, rather, occasions when they become acquainted with one another in order to enter into fugitive extra-conjugal relationships.

The members of the older generation are to-day inclined to take their tone from those of the younger, parents being afraid that they will be looked upon as utterly out of date unless they share or tolerate modern principles. The upshot has been a decline in the prevalence of a healthy and exemplary family life. Necessarily, therewith, there has ensued a marked falling off in the intellectual and artistic interests characteristic of social intercourse. Indeed, the whole field of intellectual and artistic activity has been affected for the worse. Seldom has any period in history been characterised by so complete a lack of interest in philosophy. In music, as in the other arts, the public assumes a purely passive attitude. Wireless and the films occupy eye and ear without demanding active participation. In the home and at private entertainments instrumental music and singing have now become exceptional. Bridge playing has spread like an epidemic, having become the main interest of circles where at one time the cultivation of intellect was the chief concern. The delight in genuine humour, too, seems almost to have become a thing of the past. Satire, mockery, making fun of everything, are dominant. Things are little better even in academic circles. On the whole it must be admitted that the present age has created a human type which is profoundly lacking in the power of concentration, in the power of collecting its thoughts, and which seeks " distraction " in the unrestricted pursuit of pleasure. The trend manifests itself everywhere in the loosening of conjugal ties, in the reluctance to bear children (even when potential mothers are in excellent health and in easy circumstances), and in the enfeeblement of masculine potency.

It cannot be denied that the members of the rising generation are in advance of their predecessors in respect of their bodily development, thanks to their devotion to sport. Yet in this matter, likewise, they show their tendency to excess and their lack of definite aims—even though the practice of some sport or other may have its value as a derivative for those who would otherwise be inclined to undue sexual indulgence.

The present writers are well aware that society is passing through a peculiar period of transition and transformation. History teaches us that after great wars and economic convulsions, degenerative phenomena are, during such periods of transition, especially apt to show themselves in the domain of the sexual life. In the terrible economic crisis, thanks to which the struggle for existence is daily becoming harder for us all, it may well be that sobriety is perforce following upon the mood of intoxication. Among our young folks there would seem to be trends in favour of a new disciplining of life for both sexes. A resanation is perhaps beginning. This resanation can be aided by the widest possible diffusion of sound knowledge of sexology and sexual hygiene.

CHAPTER II

Structure and Functions of the Male Reproductive Organs

The membrum virile or penis (there is no seemly vernacular name for this organ, the Chaucerian "yard" being obsolete) has three portions: a root, in the perineum between the thighs; a middle portion known as the body; and an anterior or terminal segment called the glans. At the proximal end of the glans is a rather prominent rim known as the corona glandis, and behind this rim, where it passes into the body of the penis, lies a furrow, the coronal furrow. Normally the glans penis is more or less completely covered by an extremely elastic fold of skin which is entirely devoid of fat and is easily retracted. This double fold of skin, known as the prepuce or foreskin, is continuous with the skin covering the body of the penis, and passes upward and laterally into the skin of the front of the abdomen, while on the back of the penis (the back when the organ is pendent) it passes into the skin of the scrotum, the sac containing the testicles. The foreskin sometimes leaves the glans partially exposed, but in many men, when the organ is pendent, it hides the glans completely. In this fold of skin we distinguish an external and an internal layer. The external layer resembles the skin covering other parts of the body, whereas the internal layer has, rather, the characteristics of mucous membrane. On the lower side of the organ (the posterior side when it is pendent) the foreskin is connected with the glans in the mid-line of the penis by a little fold known as the frænum præputii. In the inner layer of the foreskin and around the corona and its furrow are numerous sebaceous glands called Tyson's glands. These glands secrete a substance which, mixed with desquamated epithelial cells, tends to accumulate in the coronal furrow. It is known as the smegma of the prepuce, and has a characteristic smell. The integument of the glans is very thin, and is firmly attached to the subjacent tissues. In those men whose foreskin completely covers the glans when the penis is quiescent, this integument is moist and shiny; but when the glans is permanently exposed, either because the foreskin is short or because it has been removed by circumcision, the integument of the glans is dry and comparatively thick. For the act of copulation, for the production of the voluptuous sensation which accompanies sexual intercourse, and for the effecting of reproduction, the corpora cavernosa or erectile structures of the penis are of the utmost importance. There are three of them, one of them being medial, the corpus cavernosum urethræ, closely surrounding the anterior urethra (the tube by which the urine is evacuated and the semen ejaculated), and the others being paired, lying in front of the urethra (when the penis is pendent). These two latter are known as the corpora cavernosa penis. The terminal aperture of the urethra, called the meatus, is situated at the tip of the glans. The corpus cavernosum urethræ expands to form the main substance of the glans penis. The corpora cavernosa extend from the root of the penis beneath the pubic bone forward into the body of the penis. They consist of connective tissue having a spongy character and containing large venous spaces in its interstices. When the penis is quiescent, these contain very little blood; but whenever sexual excitement ensues, a somewhat complicated nervous and muscular mechanism gets to work, with the result that more blood flows into the corpora cavernosa than before, while the efflux of blood from them is checked, until they become strongly distended. Thereupon the penis grows hard and stiff, and, instead of hanging down, the greatly enlarged organ points forward and upward. This process is known as erection, being the necessary antecedent to the introduction of the male organ into the vagina of the female. In due course we shall have to consider disturbances of the mechanism of erection which may arise from diseases of the penis, diseases of the adjoining organs, or disorders of the process of innervation.

Now we must pass to the consideration of those parts of the male reproductive apparatus which cannot be seen without dissection. Having curved backwards in the root of the penis beneath the arch of the pubic bone, the urethra turns vertically upwards into the pelvis. Here it has separated from the corpora cavernosa, whose only function it is to make the erection of the penis possible. This proximal part of the urethra, known as the posterior urethra, is comparatively short, being only a few centimetres in length, and ends in the urinary bladder. The other two parts of the urethra are known respectively as the perineal urethra (that which lies between the thighs) and the penile urethra. The posterior urethra where it passes into the perineal urethra is surrounded by a strong sphincter muscle, subject to the control of the will but liable to relaxation as the outcome of involuntary nervous stimuli. Where the posterior urethra opens into the urinary bladder there is a less powerful bundle of muscular fibres which are not subject to voluntary control and yield to the pressure of the urine as soon as this becomes considerable. The authors are well aware that the foregoing description is not in full conformity with the demands of exact science, but experience has taught us that for lay readers the account here given of the urethra is more comprehensible than a strictly scientific one. On the hinder wall of the posterior or prostatic portion of the urethra is a small promontory projecting into its interior. This is known as the verumontanum or colliculus seminalis, which has in it a blind passage or sinus, the sinus pocularis of the prostate. The whole of this structure is sometimes termed the uterus masculinus, because it is a rudimentary structure homologous with the uterus of the female, the two deriving from the same cells of the sexually undifferentiated early embryo. On either side of the opening of this sinus into the posterior urethra is a little slit through which the semen secreted by the testicles and certain accessory glands passes into the urethra. These slits, in fact, are the terminal openings of the duct of the testicles, the vasa deferentia. The excretory ducts of the prostate, the gland surrounding the posterior urethra, open in the same region. The urine, of course, in the process of its evacuation, flows over the verumontanum. The urine enters the urinary bladder by two slit-like openings, the terminal extremities of the ureters, the ducts whereby the urine flows down from the kidneys, having been secreted by these organs and passed out by the renal tubules into the pelvis of each of these.

(The reader must not confuse the bony pelvis, consisting of the hip-bone and the sacrum, with the membranous pelvis of the kidney, the dilated upper end of the ureter.) A glance at the plate will make these various relationships more comprehensible. We hope that the reader will now have been enabled to form a clear idea of the way in which the urine secreted by the kidneys passes down the ureters into the bladder, and thence by way of the urethra into the outer world; and how the semen, whose most important constituents are formed in the testicles, passes down the vasa deferentia to enter the posterior urethra at the verumontanum or colliculus seminalis, and then to be ejaculated through the perineal and penile urethra, a channel common to the semen and to the urine. Now let us consider the testicles.

Every normal male has two testicles, which lie within the scrotum. This is a protrusion of the skin of the lower part of the belly wall, being formed by the descent of the testicles in the later months of embryonic life. Before that descent occurred, the testicles lay within the abdominal cavity on either side of the spine. At a certain stage of intra-uterine development a "genital prominence" appears on either side of the lower part of the abdomen. Subsequently these prominences fuse along the mid-line to form the scrotum, into which the testicles, right and left, descend through the respective inguinal canals. A sign of the coalescence of the two genital prominences remains throughout life in a ridge on the mid-line of the scrotum, known as the raphe. The scrotal raphe marks the line along which the right and the left genital prominences grew together.

The testis or testicle is of an ovoid shape, somewhat flattened laterally. It is of about the size of a plover's egg. Above and behind it passes into an accessory structure known as the epididymis, which forms a sort of cap to the testicle. The epididymis is prolonged into the vas deferens, the excretory duct of the testicles. Passing upwards as part of a composite structure known as the spermatic cord, it enters the abdominal cavity through the inguinal canal, and ultimately debouches, as previously described, in the posterior urethra. But before its terminal aperture is reached, there is a diverticulum, a tube leading into a blind pouch, lying on the base of the bladder, and known as the vesicula seminalis. It used to be believed that the only function of the vesiculæ seminales was to serve as reservoirs for the testicular secretion, but in actual fact these structures are independent glands, excreting an albuminous fluid having a characteristic odour. Their excretory ducts join the vasa deferentia to form a common tube, with the result that just before the outlet into the posterior urethra the secretion of the testicle is mingled with that of the vesicula seminalis. In the posterior urethra a third important element is added to the semen at the time of ejaculation. We refer to the secretion of the prostate, a gland very liable to gonorrhœal infection, and susceptible to treatment by massage or diathermy by way of the rectum (the lowest part of the bowel). Very few persons suffering from urethral and prostatic infection have any idea of the anatomical relationships of this region.

Figure 3 in Plate I shows how the prostate is situated in relation to the posterior urethra, the rectum, and the base of the bladder. It is of about the size of a walnut, and does

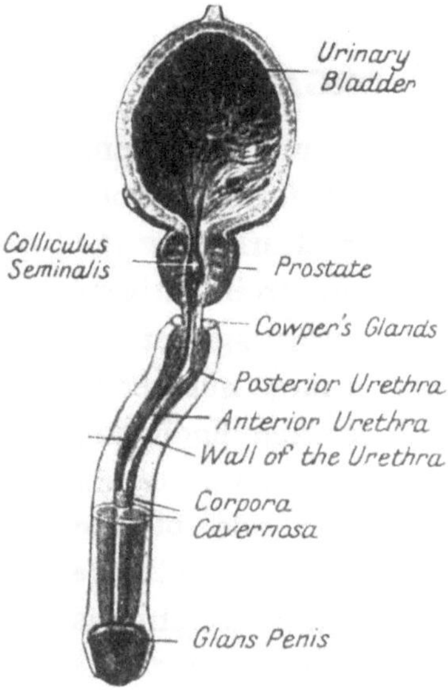

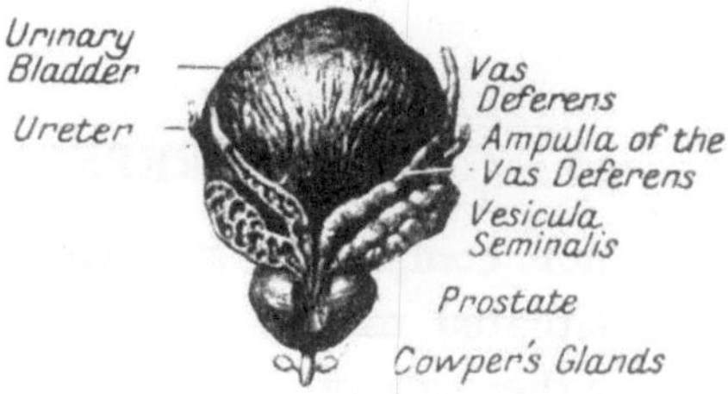

Urinary Bladder from behind

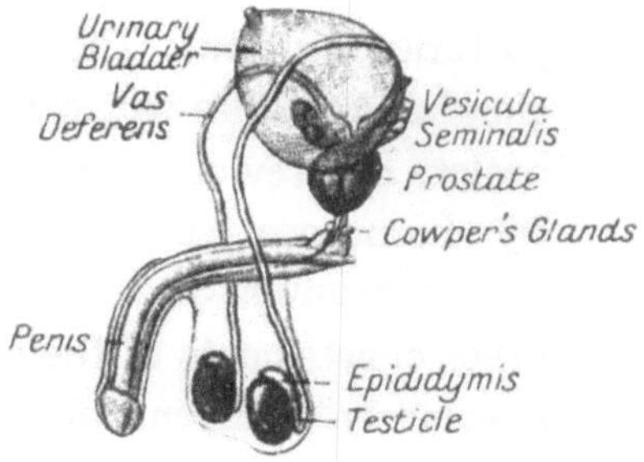

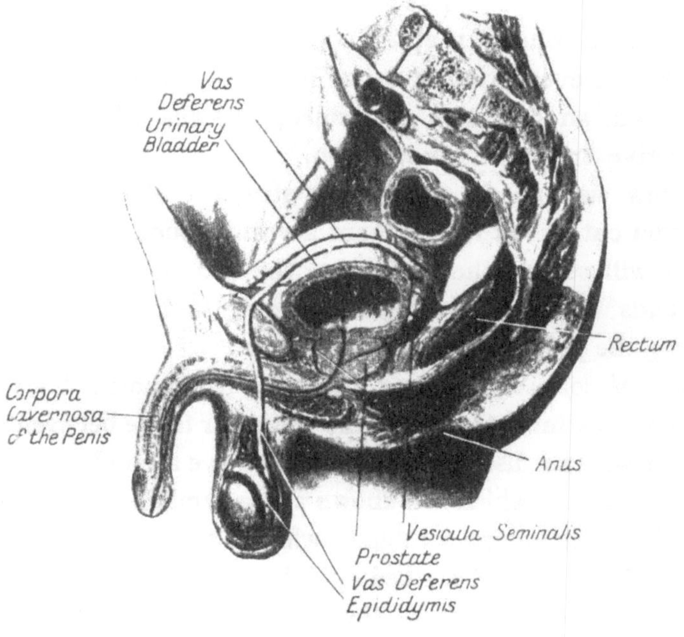

not completely surround the prostatic urethra, being situated mainly behind it, but extending forward along either side of the tube. The figure shows clearly how the surgeon's finger introduced into the rectum can investigate the back of the prostate and press it forward against the posterior urethra. The gland contains a large number of glandular tubules which form a milky secretion, finding an outlet, as previously explained, into the prostatic urethra by numerous small openings on either side of the verumontanum, and, during ejaculation, mingling with the other constituents of the semen. The prostatic secretion is absolutely indispensable to the adequate motility of the spermatozoa. We may mention in passing that in old age the prostate is liable to undergo hypertrophy and induration, when it is apt to constrict the urethra, and may make the evacuation of urine impossible unless a catheter be used, an operation performed, or some other kind of effective treatment undertaken.

Now we come to the minute structure of the testicles. If you cut one of these organs across through its long axis you will see on the surface of the section a number of strands of connective tissue forming septa, which unite along the posterior margin of the organ to constitute a thick mass of connective tissue known as Highmore's body or the mediastinum testis. In the testicular tissue between the septa we can discern with the naked eye a number of contorted canals, which are known as the seminiferous tubules. In these seminiferous tubules, which ultimately coalesce to form the already described epididymis, there is a secretion formed by their walls, this being the most important constituent of the semen. Under the microscope we find this secretion to be full of the male reproductive elements known as spermatozoa. When examined in the ejaculated semen (highly magnified) we note that they consist of an ovoid head, a neck, and a long tail which is in constant movement—a kind of whip-lash which drives the little creature rapidly hither and thither. The spermatozoa are the final product of a complicated developmental process which goes on in the cells lining the seminiferous tubules. In the quiescent state this epithelium is composed of several layers of rounded cells; but when spermatogenesis is actively going on, these cells become divided into two kinds of cells: the cells of Sertoli which form a supporting tissue; and the spermatogonia. During the period of sexual maturity, the latter are continually dividing each into two spermatocytes, primary and secondary, out of which are formed spermatids, and from these, ultimately, the spermatozoa. Between the seminiferous tubules lie groups of other cells, the interstitial cells of the testicle or Leydig's cells. Their importance as constituting what Steinach has called the "puberty gland" has, by this Austrian investigator and his disciples, been brought into the foreground of the discussion concerning rejuvenation. According to the theory propounded by Steinach, the cells of Leydig constitute an organ whose activity has a profound influence upon bodily, mental, and sexual development, while the decline of sexual powers and the onset of old age are supposed to depend mainly upon the cessation of their activity. The "puberty gland", in fact, is looked upon as one of the glands of internal secretion, one of those endocrine glands whose function it is to produce substances which are poured into the blood.

Interacting with the internal secretion of various other glands such as the adrenals and the pituitary (a small body situated at the base of the brain), the testicular hormone, as it is called, exerts a profound influence, not only upon the sexual life, but also upon the character of the individual. Other important endocrine glands, modifying nutrition, determining growth, etc., are the thyroid, and the islands of Langerhans in the pancreas (which produce insulin). We shall have occasion later to say something more about endocrinology, and shall attempt to distinguish the positive acquirements of science in this field from the products of fantasy.

In order that the reader may understand the functions of the male reproductive organs, it will be necessary for us to stress some of the anatomical details already mentioned, and to describe certain minutiæ.

The urethra, as previously said, traverses the whole length of the penis, and consists of three portions. The uppermost, the posterior urethra, lying within the pelvis, is also known as the "prostatic urethra", because it is partially enveloped by the prostate. Around the upper and the lower end of this portion are sphincter muscles, the lower one being the stronger. Downwards and forwards the urethra passes into what is known as the perineal urethra, which lies beneath the pubic bones and (in the root of the penis) is sheathed by the muscles of the perineum. The distal part of the urethra, the longest portion, is contained in the free part of the penis, which is pendent in the unexcited state, and is about 4 inches long. When erect, the penis is quasi-cylindrical in form, but flat from before backward, and in the reproductive act distends and almost completely fills the vagina of the female. Let us further reiterate that the skin of the penis is very thin, devoid of fat, and hairless ; and that it is prolonged over the coronal furrow and the glans penis into a double fold known as the foreskin or prepuce. In the preputial sac, on the middle of the lower side of the penis, there is a triangular fold of skin or membrane, the frænum præputii, passing from the foreskin to the glans. This frænum limits to some extent the retraction of the foreskin, and it corresponds to the frænum of the clitoris, which will be described in due course as part of the female reproductive organs. At this juncture it will be enough to mention that the clitoris of the female is homologous with the penis of the male, but is very much smaller. The sebaceous glands on the inner surface of the foreskin and the coronal furrow may in some persons secrete an excess of sebum (smegma), and if this is retained through insufficient retraction of the foreskin it may give rise to inflammation. Cleansing of the preputial sac and of the coronal furrow should be one of the cares of the toilet, in order to prevent such inflammation, which may extend to the skin of the glans penis producing what is called balanitis. Retention of smegma, however, is not the only cause of balanitis, which may arise in connection with the venereal diseases, or some other form of bacterial infection. This is a good place to mention that in sexually mature men there may often be seen in the preputial sac and especially along the corona glandis small thick prominences ranging from one fiftieth to one twenty-fifth of an inch in diameter. These " papillæ " are normal, not morbid, but do not appear until puberty. In certain other animals they are much larger than in man, constituting the " spines " on the penis of the

PLATE II

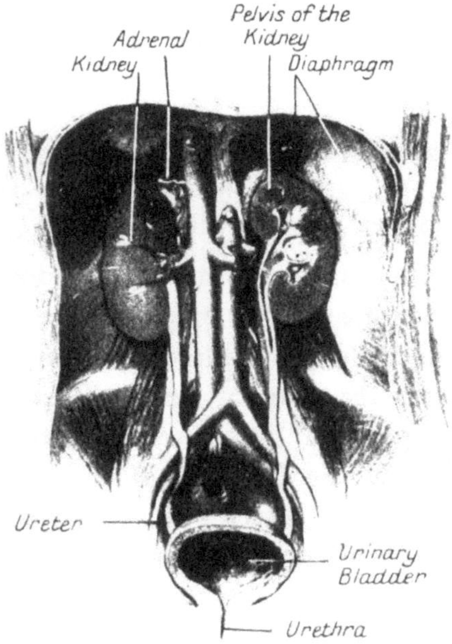

FIG. 4.—Urinary Organs, Left Kidney seen in Section*

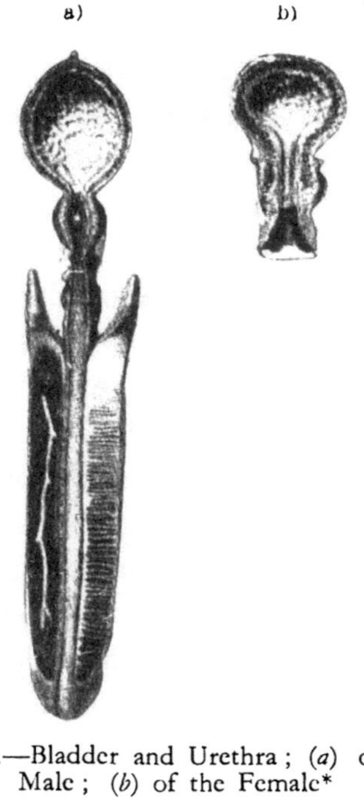

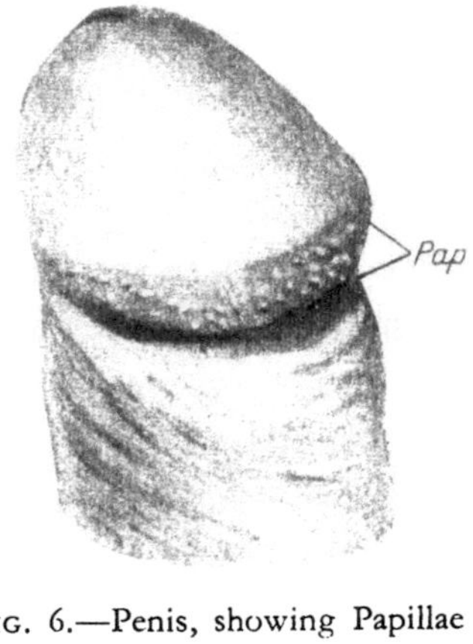

FIG. 5.—Bladder and Urethra; (*a*) of the Male; (*b*) of the Female*

FIG. 6.—Penis, showing Papillae

* (*From the Collection in the German Museum of Hygiene at Dresden*)

guinea-pig, and the dentate prominences seen on the penis of many monkeys, tom-cats, etc. The papillæ of the human male will be seen in Fig. 6, Plate II. In the human species they have no functional importance, being rudimentary, like the cæcum and the coccyx.

The skin of the penis is very richly supplied with nerves, and this remark especially concerns the glans, where there is a close-meshed network of nerve fibres with innumerable nerve terminals. Their function is to receive and transmit the sexual stimuli which, by a reflex mechanism, initiate and maintain the distension of the corpora cavernosa with blood and thus effect the erection of the penis. Erection cannot be directly produced by an act of will; it can only be brought about either by mechanical stimulation of the penis, or else by sexual images arising in the psyche. Apart from this, however, erections may occur spontaneously, as the outcome of stimuli whose causes remain obscure. They are, perhaps, dependent upon certain products of internal secretion, which, circulating in the blood, may stimulate the sexual centres in the spinal cord. Morbid inflammatory processes in the structures accessory to the penis sometimes cause erection. For instance, extremely obstinate and painful erection may occur when there is gonorrhœal inflammation of the vesiculæ seminales. Persistent and painful erections are likewise apt to occur in the disease known as leukæmia, which is characterised by an enormous increase in the white corpuscles of the blood. Long-lasting erections are also seen as a result of injuries and diseases of the spinal cord. The technical name for such enduring and purposeless erections is priapism, the term being derived from Priapus, the name of the Greek god of fruitfulness whose statues represent him with an erect penis. Localised inflammation in the corpora cavernosa, resulting from gonorrhœa, gout, arteriosclerosis, or an unknown cause, may block the inflow into some of the cavernous sinuses, so that when the penis becomes erect it is bent in one direction or another (chordee). Apart from the treatment of the primary cause (gonorrhœa, gout, etc.) some of these patients can be helped by local treatment with radium; but many cases prove incurable. During the years of sexual maturity males are apt to wake up in the morning with the penis erect, the erection being due in this case to reflex stimuli proceeding from a full bladder. Sometimes, moreover, straining at stool may cause erection, especially when the rectum contains large masses of fæces which press upon the vesiculæ seminales and upon the posterior portion of the urethra. It should further be mentioned that warmth tends to promote and cold tends to hinder erection. Extreme cold may make erection impossible even in a man who is in a condition of strong sexual excitement.

When the penis becomes erect, it is transformed from a small, pendent, and flabby organ into a much larger and elastically rigid structure, so that it is capable of penetrating the female vagina in order that, on ejaculation, the semen can be deposited at the mouth of the uterus, situate at the upper end of the vagina. The erect penis has a slight curve which corresponds precisely to the curvature of the vagina. Under normal conditions, erection is transitory, relaxation of the penis (detumescence through the emptying of the corpora cavernosa) resulting either from ejaculation or from fatigue of the erectile mechanism and diversion of the attention to other matters than sexual.

In the perineum there are paired glands known as Cowper's glands whose ducts open into the perineal portion of the urethra, and in the mucous membrane of the penile urethra there are numerous small mucous glands (the glands of Littré and the lacunæ of Morgagni). In conditions of sexual excitement, these various glands secrete a thin glairy fluid, which flows out of the urinary meatus (urethrorrhœa ex libidine). Presumably this mucous fluid serves to lubricate the penis and helps in other ways to facilitate penetration of the vagina. The ordinary reaction within the urethra is acid, owing to the acidity of the urine, but this secretion of the mucous glands of the urethra is alkaline, and therefore neutralises the urinary acid. At the same time it lubricates the interior of the urethra, thus facilitating ejaculation. In a good many men this mucous discharge from the urethra (due to sexual excitement) precedes complete erection, and persons thus affected are often alarmed thereby, regarding the urethrorrhœa as a morbid discharge of semen or as a symptom of venereal disorder. Competent medical examination will soon set their minds at rest.

When the penis becomes erect, it is four or five times as large as before. This enlargement leads mechanically to a retraction of the foreskin and an exposure of the glans. The urethra is likewise much elongated, and is transformed from a wrinkled tube into one having a smooth and frictionless interior. The distension of the corpora cavernosa which produces erection is partly due to an increased inflow of blood dependent upon a reflex dilation of the arteries supplying the penis, and partly to the contraction of certain muscles which press the principal vein of the penis (obvious on the dorsum of that organ) against the junction of the pubic bone, thus checking the outflow of blood.

When erection is complete and penetration has been effected, the to and fro movements of the male organ within the vagina produce a sort of aspiration, and the working of the reflex nervous mechanism under the stimulation of the nerve terminals in the sensitive skin of the penis causes a spasmodic contraction of the perineal and urethral muscles whereby the semen, pouring actively down the vasa deferentia and mingled in the posterior urethra with secretions of the vesiculæ seminales and the prostate, is explosively ejaculated into the vagina, to the accompaniment of the climax of voluptuous sensation known as the orgasm. At this moment the sexual excitement extends to the whole body in so far as it is subject to the dominion of that part of the nervous system which is called " autonomic ", this meaning independent, as contrasted with the part of the nervous system subject to voluntary control. The pupils enlarge, the skin reddens, the heart beats more frequently and more potently, the breathing is likewise quickened, moderate sweating occurs, and there are reflex, cramp-like extensions of the limbs. After the orgasm comes complete relaxation, the tension suddenly passing off, being usually succeeded by fatigue and a need for sleep. In a good many men the sudden transition from extreme sexual tension to complete relaxation is accompanied by a feeling of depression, which may be melancholic in its intensity. The relaxation affects the internal organs likewise, and leads in quite a number of

PLAITE III

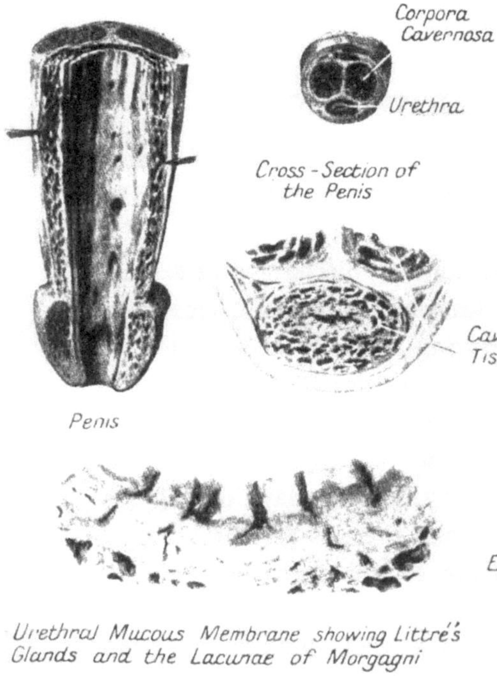

FIG. 7.—Mucous Membrane of the Male Urethra

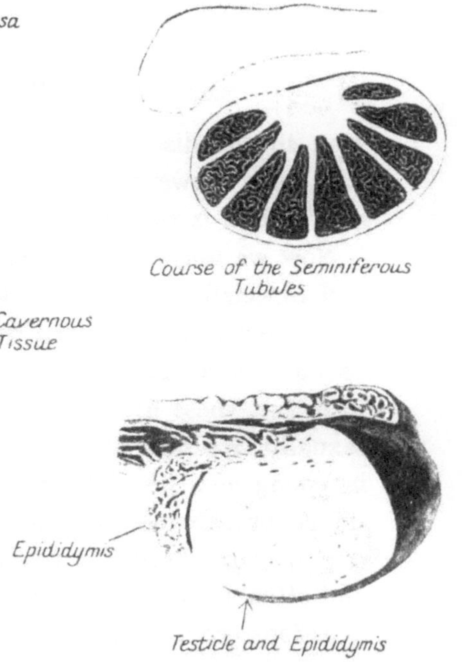

FIG. 8.—Structure of the Testicle

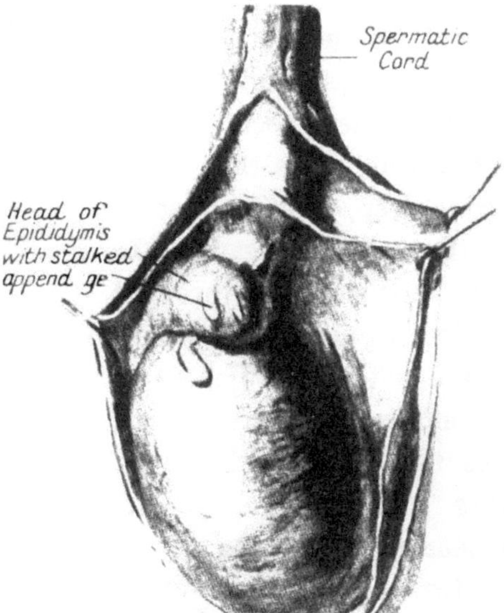

FIG. 9.—Right Testicle and Epididymis, seen from the left, the Tunics having been slit open

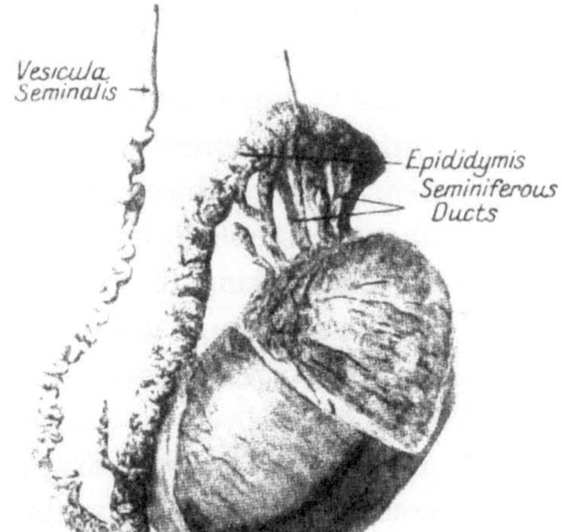

FIG. 10.—Right Testicle (a part has been cut away) and Epididymis freed from the Tunics

(From the Collection in the German Museum of Hygiene at Dresden)

men to the discharge of very large quantities of urine. Ere long, however, a condition of mental and bodily equilibrium is re-established.

Now we must refer to involuntary discharges of semen, and especially to what are known as nocturnal emissions (the ejaculation of semen during sleep or a condition of partial awakening), since it is important to emphasise the fact that these are nowise morbid. They may occur in sexually ripe men at any age, but are especially frequent in young men just after puberty, taking place during the small hours of the morning, when there is a summation of stimuli from distended vesiculæ seminales, a full bladder, and often a full rectum. Almost invariably such nocturnal emissions occur at the climax of a voluptuous dream, from which the sleeper partially awakens as ejaculation occurs. In men who are sexually competent and who are living an abstinent life it is perfectly normal for such a nocturnal emission to occur every week or ten days. Involuntary ejaculations are only morbid when they occur before puberty, when they are unduly frequent, when they occur in the waking state instead of during sleep, or are connected with some abnormal state of the genital organs. In neurasthenic subjects, morbid ejaculations may be brought about by the slight friction of the clothing against the penis; by the shaking to which one is inevitably subjected in a railway train, a tramcar, or a motor-car; when riding or doing gymnastics. Sometimes they may occur as an outcome of voluptuous thoughts. Morbid, too, is the discharge of a few drops of semen in the absence of erection. In concluding this chapter we may mention that in connection with the sudden death of a man in his sexual prime, and especially in persons executed by hanging, ejaculation often occurs in the death agony. The medieval legends about mandragora (which was supposed to grow with special luxuriance beneath the gallows) and about its influence in promoting fertility are the expression of this physiological fact.

CHAPTER III

The Semen

The semen, the normal ejaculation of the sexually ripe male, is a viscid, sticky fluid having a milky and vitreous appearance. Chemically it is composed of various albumins and of the fat-like substances known as lecithin, mucin, and cholesterin. Soon after the ejaculation of the semen, crystals of the substance called spermin form in the fluid. This spermin is said to give the ejaculated semen its typical odour of herrings. Von Pöhl, a Petrograd investigator, found that spermin has a stimulating action upon metabolism (tissue change). Van de Velde thinks it is not improbable that the absorption of spermin from the vagina may exert a tonic influence upon woman. This question, however, must be left open. All that we certainly know about spermin is that it is not derived from the secretion of the testicles. We find, indeed, that we can obtain more spermin crystals from an ejaculation which is comparatively poor in spermatozoa.

In the human semen there are about sixty million spermatozoa in each cubic centimetre, so that in a normal ejaculation, which amounts to from three to eight cubic centimetres, there may be as many as five hundred million spermatozoa. Enough was said in the previous chapter about the complicated and lengthy process of development whereby the spermatozoa arise out of certain cells lining the seminiferous tubules. The length of the finished spermatozoon, consisting of head, neck, and tail, ranges from five to six thousandths of a millimetre. Looked at from above, the head is elliptical, but seen from the side it is somewhat pear-shaped. In the testicle the spermatozoa are motionless and are presumably passed on from the testicle proper to the epididymis by the contraction of involuntary muscular fibres. In the epididymis the tubules a lined with what is known as ciliated epithelium, this meaning that the cells have protrusions like whip-lashes which wave continually towards the outlet. Fluid elements are added to the secretion in the epididymis, and by the movements of the cilia and the contraction of involuntary muscular fibres the onward progress of the semen is effected. In the course of their passage along the vasa deferentia, the spontaneous movements of the spermatoza begin. In the urethra, during the act of ejaculation, the testicular secretion is mingled with the secretion from the prostate, which, as already said, greatly intensifies the motility of the spermatozoa.

The vesiculæ seminales (which are lacking in many mammals) must not be regarded as mere reservoirs for the semen, for their lining mucous membrane contributes its own peculiar secretion to the semen. This secretion is still formed when the vasa deferentia have been ligatured or have been blocked by inflammation or when the persons concerned have been castrated. The secretion of the lining cells of the vesiculæ seminales is a viscid, yellowish substance, which is probably one of the main causes of the peculiar stickiness of the ejaculated semen. The stickiness is transient, disappearing when the little lumps (like sago grains) contributed by the vesiculæ seminales have been

PLATE IV

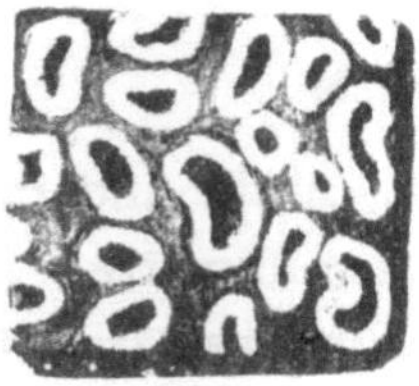

Section of a Lobe of the Testicle

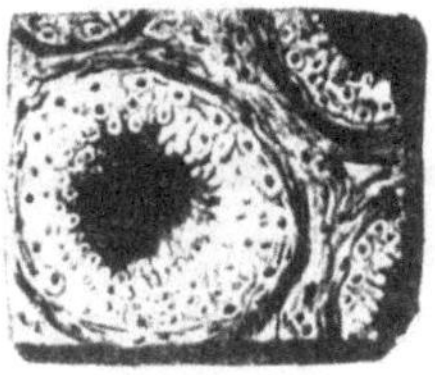

Seminiferous Tubules seen in Cross-Section

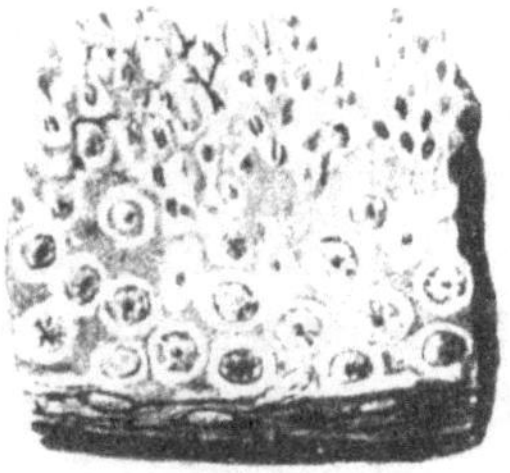

Section of the Wall of a Convoluted Seminiferous Tubule

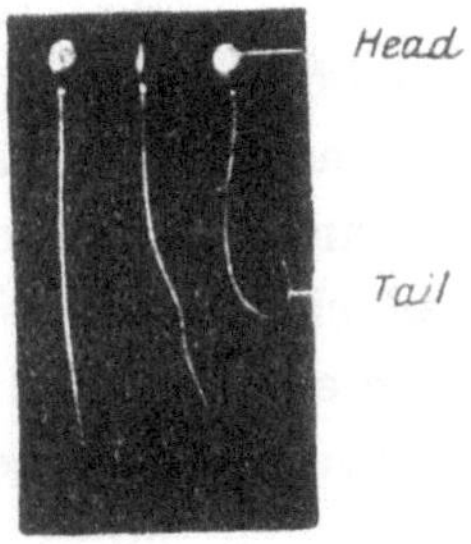

Spermatozoa

FIGS. 11 TO 14.—Minute structure of the Testicle

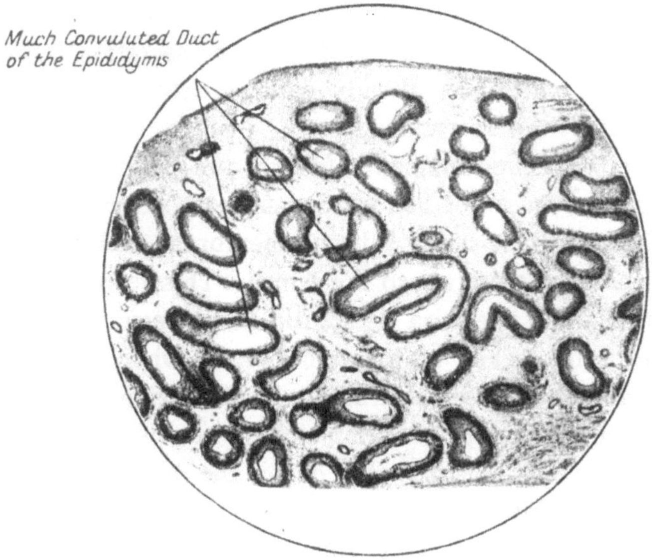

FIG. 15.—Magnified Section of the Epididymis

(From the Collection in the German Museum of Hygiene at Dresden)

broken up and dissolved in the semen. We do not really know what importance the secretion of the vesiculæ seminales has. Many authors believe that it may activate the spermatozoa in some way. Others consider that the main function of the vesicles is to serve as supplementary reservoirs for the testicular secretion, which is normally stored up in the seminal ampullæ, thimble-shaped expansions of the vasa deferentia.

The prostate consists of from thirty to fifty glandular tubules, and of considerable quantities of involuntary muscular fibres which can expel the prostatic secretion into the urethra. The prostatic musculature is interconnected with the involuntary muscular tissues coating the vesiculæ seminales, so that, during ejaculation, the prostatic duct and the vesiculæ seminales are simultaneously emptied into the posterior urethra. The normal prostatic secretion has a milky aspect. In addition to albuminous and fatty substances, it contains corpuscles of neutral calcium phosphate which concrete around desquamated epithelial cells, and are known as corpora amylacea. The prostatic secretion dilutes the semen and promotes the motility of the spermatozoa. It would seem, moreover, that the peculiar smell of semen is dependent upon the admixture with prostatic secretion, and if so we may presume that spermin is derived from the prostate. At ordinary times the secretion of the prostate is scanty, but under the influence of sexual ideas and stimuli it can increase to an enormous extent.

It will be seen, then, that the semen as ejaculated is an extremely composite fluid, containing, in addition to the spermatozoa and the fluid produced in the testicle proper, elements contributed by the epididymis, the seminal vesicle, the prostate, Cowper's gland, and the mucous glands of the anterior urethra.

The internal secretion of the male reproductive glands, the "hormones" poured into the blood as contrasted with the external secretions which form the ejaculated semen, is of the utmost importance to the mental and bodily equilibrium of the male, to his working powers and general functional capacity, and above all to his inclination to make sexual advances towards a possible reproductive partner. At puberty, when the testicles "ripen", not only does the secretion of the semen begin, but at the same time, with the formation of the sexual hormones, there occurs the transformation of the boy into the young man. When the testicles begin to grow old, when there is a marked decline in the amount of their incretion, the body (and often the mind as well) begins to show signs of age. Upon their activity depends the appearance of the secondary sexual characters, namely, the specifically masculine development of the bones and the muscles, the "breaking" of the voice, the growth of the beard, etc. We cannot go into details regarding some of the more debatable problems of endocrinology, but may mention, in concluding this chapter, that certain investigators consider that the development of masculine secondary sexual characters is not exclusively due to the hormones produced by the testicle, believing that those produced by the epididymis, the prostate, and the seminal vesicle contribute.

CHAPTER IV

Anatomy of the Female Reproductive Organs

In women as in men we have to distinguish between the external and the internal reproductive organs. In the male the urethra is the common excretory duct for the urine and for the semen. In woman the labia majora and minora conceal the separate openings of the urinary passage and the vagina, which lie within the vulval cleft. (See Fig. 16, Plate V.) The labia majora are two large folds of skin covered with a growth of stiff hair and richly supplied with sebaceous glands. In young girls and in virgins of more advanced years they lie in very close apposition, but the vulval cleft often gapes a little in married women, especially in those who have borne children. On the lower part of the belly wall, immediately in front of and above the anterior junction of the labia majora, is a prominence formed by a pad of fat beneath the skin which in sexually mature women is thickly covered with hair—the pubic hair. This prominence is known as the mons veneris. Below and behind, the labia majora are likewise connected by a fold of skin situated in front of the anus. Within the labia majora lie the smaller folds known as the labia minora, which join in the mid-line in front, their anterior ends splitting to surround the clitoris which, as already said, is homologous with the penis, but much smaller, and not (as in the male) traversed by the urethra. The inferior opening of that canal lies a little way behind the clitoris, and still farther back we see, in virgins, the membrane known as the hymen. This varies in shape, but is most often a semilunar fold of mucous membrane continuous at the apex and in front with the mucous membrane covering the labia minora. Normally it is pierced by a central opening, the vaginal orifice, but in occasional instances it is cribriform (containing numerous small openings instead of one large one); and in rare cases there is no opening at all (imperforate hymen). The hymen is torn in the first act of sexual intercourse, and the remnants of the torn membrane atrophy until nothing is left but small vestigial prominences known as the carunculæ myrtiformes. The hymen is peculiar to the human species, not being found in the closely related anthropoid apes. Paired glands, called Bartholin's glands, lie beneath the mucous membrane on either side of the vaginal inlet. These glands produce a mucous secretion which becomes much more profuse under conditions of sexual excitement, serving to lubricate the vaginal inlet and facilitate penetration. There are also sebaceous glands scattered along the inner surfaces of the labia minora.

Whereas the male urethra is about 8 inches long, the female urethra is much shorter, being little more than an inch in length. Inwardly it opens into the urinary bladder just beneath the arch of the pubic bones. As we see in Plate V, the vagina (the lower part of the female reproductive canal) lies behind and below the urethra. It is a membranous passage, partially closed in virgins at its outer end by the hymen, while the neck or cervix of the womb or uterus projects into its upper end. In the middle of the cervix is an aperture, the mouth of the womb or os uteri. Thus the upper end of the vagina forms a sort

PLATE V

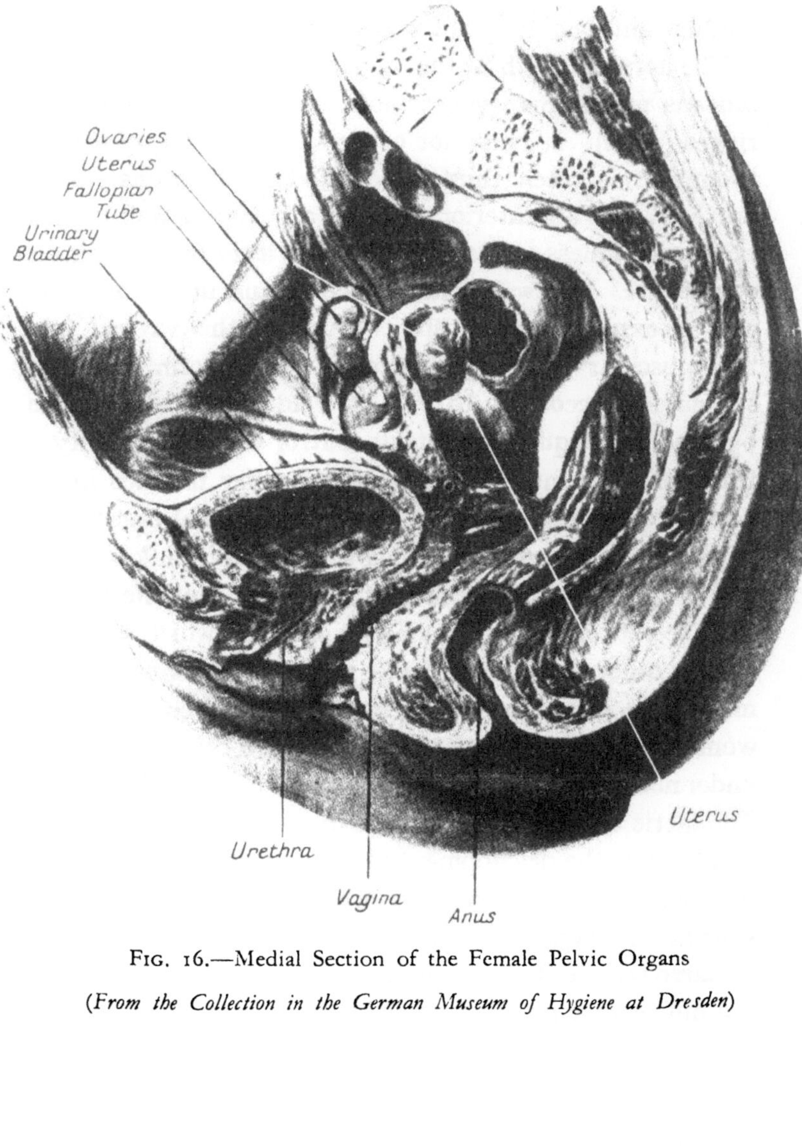

FIG. 16.—Medial Section of the Female Pelvic Organs

(From the Collection in the German Museum of Hygiene at Dresden)

of arch (fornix) into which the neck of the uterus projects, the part of the arch in front of the neck being called the anterior fornix and the part behind the neck the posterior fornix. In front of the vagina are the urethra and the bladder and behind it is the rectum.

The normal length of the vagina is about 3½ inches. The mucous membrane lining it exhibits numerous transverse ridges (rugæ). It must not be considered as an open tube, though it is often thus represented in diagrams. It is flattened, has an anterior wall and a posterior wall in close apposition unless artificially separated, as in the act of intercourse, etc. The wall contains elastic and muscular fibres, and is extremely distensible. Around the vaginal inlet the muscular fibres are concentrated to form a sort of sphincter. According to Van de Velde, some women can, by practice, acquire voluntary control over the activity of this sphincter muscle and over the other muscles in the pelvic floor which are concerned in the sexual orgasm.

The mucous membrane lining the vagina is pink in colour and is rather thin. It contains no glands, but the mucous cells secrete a moderate amount of fluid which contains, among other ingredients, lactic acid. The vaginal mucous membrane is not germ-free, but always, even in healthy women, gives hospitality to various micro-organisms which, under normal conditions, are not merely harmless but useful. The lactic acid favours the growth of the useful organisms and hinders the development of pathogenic organisms liable to cause catarrh and other forms of inflammation. In ageing women the vagina gradually becomes inelastic; its canal is narrowed, and the walls are thinner than they were; the mucous membrane is atrophied and sometimes fissured.

The length, calibre, and extensibility of the vagina vary much, however, not only in accordance with age, but also in accordance with the number of times the woman concerned has been pregnant.

The womb or uterus is an organ composed mainly of muscle, and having approximately the size and shape of a small pear. We have already described how its lower part, or cervix, projects downwards into the vaginal fornix. The remainder of the uterus, known as the body, lies within the abdominal cavity. The womb is a hollow structure, its mouth opening, as aforesaid, through the cervix into the fornix of the vagina. The cavity of the body of the uterus is flat from before backwards and expands at the upper end laterally so as to form a triangle, and into the two upper angles of this triangle open the oviducts or Fallopian tubes down which the ova pass into the interior of the uterus. At the upper end, the Fallopian tubes form on either side a trumpet-shaped expansion which opens freely into the abdominal cavity. The expanded, trumpet-shaped end exhibits ridges known as fimbriæ (see Plate V). The aspect is somewhat like that of a fibrillated root, and it has a considerable resemblance to the plant known as Scabiosa morsus diaboli. For this reason, the anatomists of an earlier day, who were botanists in summer-time, called the fimbriated extremity of the Fallopian tubes "morsus diaboli". Although the oviduct is not directly continuous with the ovary, its abdominal aperture is closely adjacent to this gland, with the result that—normally—when an ovum is discharged from the ovary it passes into the Fallopian tube, to be fertilised there, or (should fertilisation fail to occur) to pass on into the uterus and to be ejected from the body. In very rare instances, the ovum "misses its mark" so to say, and gets loose in the abdominal cavity instead of being shot into the Fallopian tube. Since the spermatozoa can, through the Fallopian tubes, gain access to the abdominal cavity, such an ovum may be fertilised, and an extra-uterine pregnancy may result. A more common form of the justly dreaded extra-uterine pregnancy is that which ensues when an ovum, having been fertilised in the tube, fails to make its way down into the cavity of the uterus. To this matter of "tubal pregnancy" we shall return.

The female reproductive glands, the ovaries, are, like the testicles, two in number. Each of them is a flattened, ovoid body, ranging in length from 1 to 2 inches, from ¾ in. to a little more than an inch in width, and in thickness from ⅛ in. to ⅜ in. Their position on either side of the uterus in close proximity to the fimbriated extremity of the Fallopian tubes can be gathered from a study of Figs. 17 and 18 in Plate VI. In the interior of the ovary are its essential reproductive elements which in the earliest stage of their development are known as the primordial follicles. These primordial follicles already exist in the ovaries of the new-born girl, as tiny sacs surrounded by a wall or theca consisting of several layers of cells and containing a dense fluid in its interior in which the ovum or egg-cell floats. At puberty these primordial follicles increase notably in size, and whenever one of them ripens it tends to project from the rounded surface of the ovary. When they have reached a certain degree of ripeness the follicles are spoken of as Graafian follicles. The ovum within the Graafian follicles is no larger than a grain of sand, being just visible to the naked eye. Its minute structure has been learned by the use of the microscope. It consists of a white shining transparent envelope, the zona pellucida ; a cavity filled with lymph ; and a granular protoplasm or yelk. Prominent within this is the germinal vehicle or nucleus, in which, under high powers of the microscope, can be seen a tiny corpuscle, the nucleolus. Just as the spermatozoa develop out of the testicular cells, so do the ova develop out of the cells of the ovary, passing through an intermediate stage in which the cells are called ovogonia. From puberty onwards, throughout the period of active sexual life, there ensues every four weeks a congestive enlargement of the right ovary or the left (alternately) with an enlargement of the ovum in the Graafian follicle which happen to be ripening.

The primordial follicles make their appearance in the ovary at a comparatively early stage of intra-uterine life, and at birth the new-born female infant has within her round about forty thousand such follicles. Only a small proportion of these ripen to become Graafian follicles, and they do not become capable of fertilisation before puberty, which in the European races and in temperate climes occurs at about the age of 14. The process of complete ripening of a Graafian follicle is known as ovulation. At the climax, the follicles burst and the ovum passes into the Fallopian tube. Thereafter the cells of the collapsed follicles develop into an organ of the utmost functional importance, the corpus luteum (yellow body).

The Fallopian tube or oviduct is lined with ciliated mucous membrane (see above), the cilia waving persistently towards the uterus, and gradually sweeping the ovum down the tube. The passage through the tube is supposed to take

PLATE VI

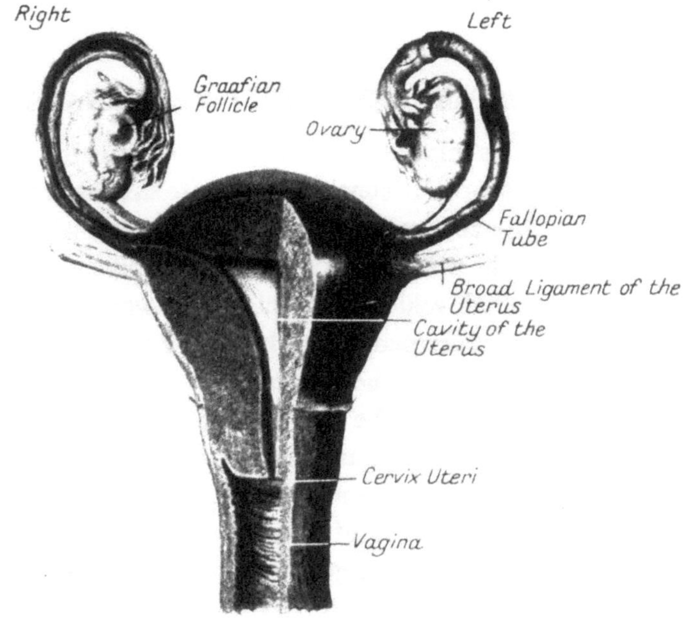

FIG. 17.—Internal Female Reproductive Organs, the Right Anterior Part of the Uterine Wall having been cut away

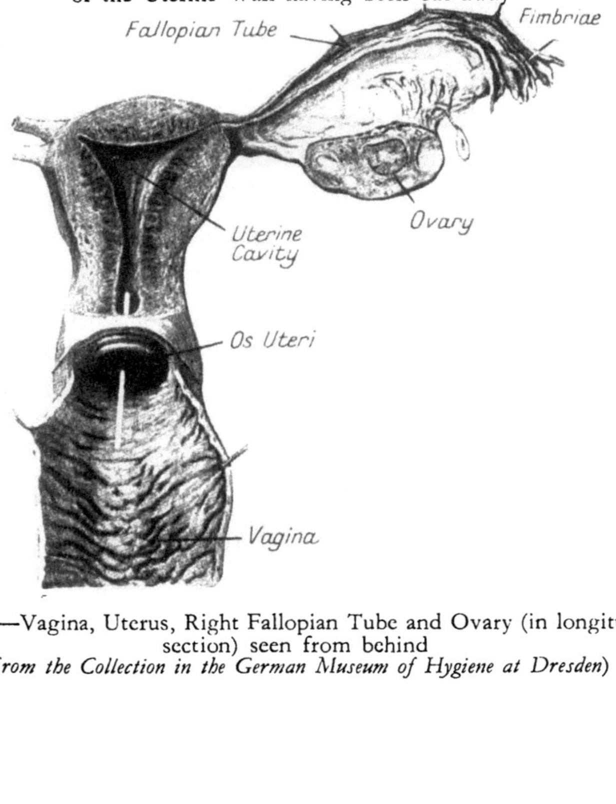

FIG. 18.—Vagina, Uterus, Right Fallopian Tube and Ovary (in longitudinal section) seen from behind
(*From the Collection in the German Museum of Hygiene at Dresden*)

about three days. The ripening of an ovum, its expulsion into the Fallopian tube, and the formation of the corpus luteum are closely connected with the periodic discharge of blood from the uterus which, from puberty to the climacteric, occurs in normal women at regular intervals of about four weeks. The mucous membrane lining the uterus thickens, softens, and breaks down, the intra-uterine cells mixed with blood from the torn capillaries being discharged through the vaginal outlet—a process known as menstruation. The occurrence of menstruation is a sign that an ovum, ripened and discharged into the Fallopian tube ten days to a fortnight earlier, has not been fertilised. By the renovation of its lining membrane the uterus makes itself ready again and ever again for the reception of a fertilised ovum.

The average duration of the menstrual flow is about four days; the regeneration of the mucous membrane occupies from five to ten days; and the preliminaries to the menstrual desquamation take about the same time. Thus even when menstruation is in abeyance, important tissue changes are going on within the uterus. For a long time it has been generally believed that there must be a close interconnection between menstruation, ovulation, and the feminine sexual characteristics in general. We now know as a positive fact that the ovaries produce the feminine sexual hormones just as the testicles produce the sexual hormones of the male. Recent researches have proved that in women the sexual hormones originate in the cells that lined the wall of the Graafian follicle prior to its collapse. There is a complicated interaction between the activities of the corpus luteum and those of other endocrine glands—

a matter which will be more fully discussed at a later stage. Sufficient at this juncture to note that the periodical changes in the mucous membrane of the uterus, culminating month by month in the menstrual bleeding, are brought about by the action of the ovarian hormones.

During pregnancy the mammary glands or breasts begin to secrete milk; and after the birth of the child, under normal and healthy conditions, the secretion becomes far more abundant, and the mother gives suck to her infant for many months. In various other ways, moreover, the breasts are intimately connected with a woman's sexual life, and they therefore merit description. Situated on front of the chest and extending from the third to the fifth rib, the breasts consist, in both sexes, of a stratum of fatty tissue beneath the skin, under which lies a firm layer of connective tissue. Until puberty this connective-tissue mass, the mammary gland, is rudimentary in both sexes. At puberty, however, in females the breast becomes greatly enlarged, chiefly through an increase in its fatty elements. Even in males the complete atrophy of the mammary gland does not begin until the age of thirty. In the middle of the breast, both in men and in women, projects the nipple. It is darkly pigmented, and is surrounded by a pigmented circle of skin known as the areola. The lacteal function does not develop in a woman until she becomes pregnant. When this occurs, the gland cells become turgid with fat drops, which, together with albuminous substances, salts, etc., being discharged into the lacteal duct, constitute the milk. The milk first secreted during pregnancy contains, instead of the fine fat droplets of the later milk, large fatty epithelial cells, known as colostrum corpuscles, which give the secretion a peculiar yellow tinge. This early milk (colostrum) is replaced by normal milk within a few days of the birth of the child. In the new-born infant the mammary gland sometimes secretes a milky fluid, produced by a fatty change in the gland cells ; and in very exceptional instances the same thing occurs in adult males. Such a secretion is spoken of as " witches' milk ".

CHAPTER V

Menstruation and the Ovarian Cycle

It is now desirable to consider menstruation and the ovarian cycle in fuller detail. In old days it was believed that the purpose of menstruation was to cleanse the female body of certain residues. Another theory was that menstruation effected the elimination of substances which the female body had need of only during pregnancy—in order to supply materials for the growth of the child. Influenced by these erroneous views, our forefathers supposed there must be some sort of connection between the discharge of blood from the uterus after childbirth, on the one hand, and the full development of the lacteal secretion on the other. They thought that the discharge of blood in childbed must effect the elimination of substances which would otherwise be harmful to the mother. As soon as the lacteal secretion became fully established, these substances found another outlet, and the discharge of blood dried up. If both channels of exit were blocked, the noxious substances settled in one of the internal organs and gave rise to disease. Thus it was that in the days before the study of bacteriology began and before anything was known of the need for the use of antiseptics in midwifery, "puerperal fever"—the peritonitis which decimated women in childbed—was ascribed to the "striking inwards" of substances which ought to have been discharged in the milk or in the postpartum uterine flux.

Puerperal insanity, again, the acute mental disorder which sometimes ensues after childbirth, was believed to be due to a " displacement " of milk to the brain. Such theories held sway among doctors as well as laymen for about two thousand years. As Fritsch aptly remarks, they had one great advantage. They were plausible, and " plausibility often contributes much more than proof to the diffusion of a doctrine "

We know to-day that menstruation is only the outward and visible sign or accompaniment of a hidden process brought to light by the careful investigation of numerous scientists during the last eighty years, namely ovulation. Let us enlarge upon what has been said already concerning this matter.

Menstruation usually begins at the age of 13 or 14, and is an indication of approaching sexual maturity (puberty). The total quantity of the menstrual discharge in any one period ranges roughly from three to seven fluid ounces; but many authorities speak of much smaller quantities as usual, regarding about a tablespoonful as the normal daily amount, and a total quantity of more than three or four tablespoonfuls as excessive. There can be no doubt that menstruating women are inclined to exaggerate the amount of blood they lose. Still, as long as the discharge is not profuse enough for the blood to form clots, there is no reason to regard it as abnormally profuse. The usual periodicity of menstruation is a four-weekly one, approximately—the actual number of days ranging, in women who are " regular ", from twenty-six to thirty days. While the menarche (the commencement of menstruation) usually occurs in this part of the world during the fourteenth year of life, there are, as previously indicated, great differences in women of diverse races and inhabiting various climes. Among the Eskimos, for instance, women seldom menstruate at all during the long polar night, and in them the menarche occurs very late, somewhere about the twenty-third year. In the tropics, women begin to menstruate much earlier, at the age of 11 or even before. Racial differences, as well as climate, play their part in this matter. In Hungary, for instance, menstruation usually begins in the thirteenth year of life among Jewish women, and in the fifteenth year among the Magyars. Diet, and the mode of life in general, have their effect, so that among the comparatively well to do, who are richly fed, lead sedentary lives, and are intellectually more active, menstruation tends to begin earlier than among girls of the poorer classes, who are often insufficiently fed, live under bad hygienic conditions, and have to do physical work when still quite young. There are great variations in the duration of the menstrual flow as between one woman and another. In general it lasts from three to five days, but we find women who menstruate only for a day or two, and others who menstruate habitually for a week, without having to be regarded as morbid. In any particular woman, moreover, the duration of menstruation may vary with changes in climate, as a result of mental excitement, or in accordance with the state of their health. The flow usually lasts longer and is more profuse if a woman engages in active bodily exercise while menstruating. If menstruation lasts habitually less than two days or more than a week, medical examination is desirable to ascertain whether there is any other sign of morbid changes in the ovaries or the uterus.

Although the incretion of the corpus luteum is the main factor in regulating the periods, mental stimuli play a considerable part, being able in some cases to bring on menstruation before it is due, and in others to cause transient amenorrhœa (non-appearance of the flow).

At the outset of a normal menstruation, the blood is mixed with a considerable quantity of mucus, but becomes more sanguineous in the course of the flow, while towards the end it is serous and only lightly tinged with blood. The discharge has a characteristic odour, which varies in strength in different women, but is sometimes so strong that even in those who are scrupulous about cleanliness the fact that they are menstruating is obvious to anyone with a keen nose. With the onset of menstruation the uterus and the whole genital tract becomes engorged with blood. The vaginal mucous membrane is reddened; the labia are slightly swelled; a sense of weight in the lower belly, accompanied by a frequent desire to make water and an inclination to go to stool, together with aching in the lower part of the back, makes the woman aware that she is about to be "unwell". The enlargement of the breasts which occurs a few days before menstruation shows that reactions in organs which, though remote, have intimate connection with the pelvic reproductive organs, form a part of the menstrual cycle. But although the menstrual flow occurs during that part of the cycle when the uterus is most strongly congested, in quite a number of women during the intermenstrual period when the uterus is conspicuously uncongested there may for a day or two be a slight discharge of blood from the interior of the organ, accompanied by pains in the pelvis (Mittelschmerz, or periodic intermenstrual pain). Furthermore, in connection with menstruation there occur general disturbances of mind and body, usually slight but varying in degree, as an indication that all the woman's organs and functions are involved in the process of menstruation. Uncertainty of temper, lassitude and undue liability to fatigue, a marked disinclination for work, and a tendency to headache which may culminate in a definite attack of migraine, are frequently noted. There is also increased secretion of saliva. Women affected with gallstones are apt to suffer from attacks of biliary colic during the period. These arise in connection with the congestion of the liver which accompanies menstruation. Gastro-intestinal disturbances are likewise frequent: diarrhœa or constipation; nausea and vomiting; a furred tongue and a foul breath; flatulence. Shooting pains in the arms and legs sometimes become neuralgic in their intensity, and in women thus affected many of the nerve trunks will be found unduly sensitive to pressure. Disturbances of vision and of hearing have also been described. All these disorders when moderate in degree can be regarded as not transcending the limits of the normal; but when menstruation is attended by intense uterine pain or when the bleeding is extremely profuse and prolonged, the condition must be considered morbid. In the majority of such cases there is something abnormal about the position of the uterus or its appendages (the ovaries and the Fallopian tubes). Especially to be pitied are those women in whom the first hours of the period are marked by the occurrence of uterine pain which may rival labour pains in intensity. There is no panacea for such

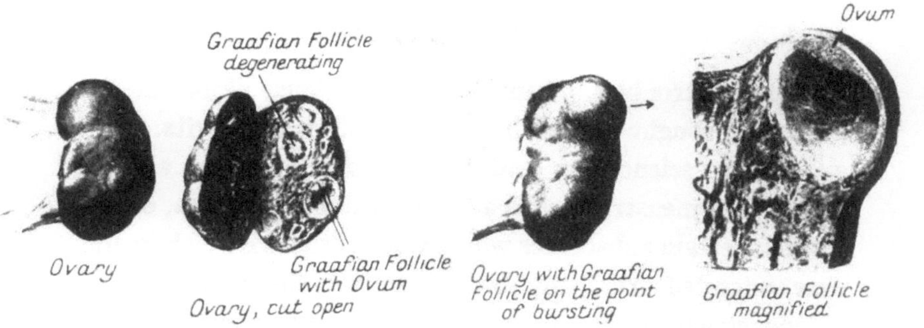

FIG. 19.—The Ovaries, the Female Reproductive Glands

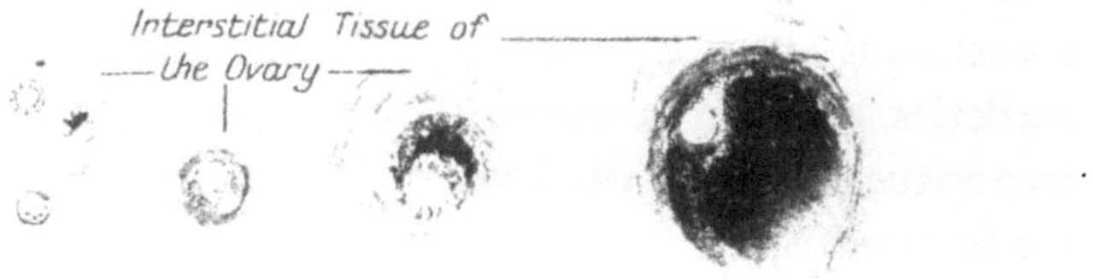

FIG. 20.—Development of the Graafian Follicle in the Ovary

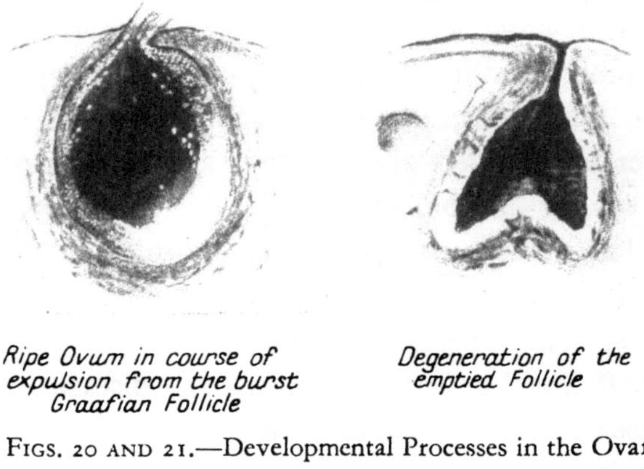

FIGS. 20 AND 21.—Developmental Processes in the Ovary

(From the Collection in the German Museum of Hygiene at Dresden)

menstrual troubles. Their causes are various. Skilled advice must be sought and each case treated on its merits.

Modern science can find no justification for the ancient view that menstruation is a "purificatory" process, one in which certain substances which would otherwise be harmful are excreted from the body; or for the view that if a menstruating woman handles cut flowers they will fade more quickly than usual, and if she kneads dough the bread will not rise.

In our latitudes menstruation usually ceases when a woman is about 49 years old. Fritsch gives the following statistics as regards the onset of what is known as the menopause: in 45 per cent of women it occurs between the forty-fifth and the fiftieth year; in 13·5 per cent before the fortieth year; in 5 per cent before the thirtieth year; in 1·8 per cent after the fiftieth year. The cessation of the periods, like their first onset, is, as regards the age at which it occurs, partly dependent upon race and diet. In eastern Germany menstruation begins on the average earlier than in the western part of the country. In virgins and in married women who have never borne children, menstruation usually ceases earlier than in women who have been mothers. More especially is the menopause apt to occur late in women who have given birth to a child after attaining the age of 40. Morbid changes in the uterus sometimes lead to a late menopause. When such morbid conditions are successfully treated, menstruation may suddenly disappear, never to return. The menopause may also be deferred in women suffering from other than uterine diseases, such as heart disease, kidney disease, emphysema, asthma, and hæmorrhoids. In this connection mention must be made of "pseudomenstruation", a bleeding from the uterine mucous membrane which may occur even in elderly women in consequence of various infections and of disturbances of the circulation. These casual hæmorrhages are not, like true menstruation, the sequel of ovulation. It was the discovery of the ovarian cycle which first gave a clue to the real nature of menstruation.

Let us, then, consider somewhat more closely this ovario-uterine cycle, which is anatomical as well as functional. After the close of each menstrual period it is only for a few days that the uterine mucous membrane retains the typical aspect of a quiescent mucous membrane. A fortnight after menstruation another Graafian follicle has ripened and burst, shooting the ovum into the expanded extremity of the Fallopian tube. Simultaneously the uterine mucous membrane becomes thickened, it secretes more mucus, the uterine bloodvessels become expanded and tortuous: in a word, we have, though in a lesser degree, the changes that occur in the pregnant uterus. Unmistakably the womb has prepared itself for the reception of a fertilised ovum. The cause of these remarkable changes in the uterine mucous membrane is the incretion of the corpus luteum formed in the ovary out of the lining cells of the Graafian follicle after the discharge of the ovum. The hormone thus produced, carried to the uterus by the blood, induces the specific changes above described. Only when the ovum has been fertilised does the corpus luteum persist in the ovary for a considerable time and go on developing as the "corpus luteum of pregnancy". Should fertilisation fail to occur, the "corpus luteum of menstruation" undergoes rapid atrophy, so that within a few days no trace of it remains in the ovary other than a small scar. The specific hormone which has caused the changes in the uterus is no longer poured into the blood. Furthermore, since fertilisation has not occurred, the changes in the uterine mucous membrane which prepared it for the reception of a fertilised ovum no longer have any meaning. The mucous membrane atrophies, like the corpus luteum of menstruation; it desquamates, its capillaries are torn across, and nothing remains but mucus, blood, and shreds of tissue, which the uterus has to discharge from its interior. Being a muscular organ, the womb contracts and expels the debris, which flows out of the vagina as the menstrual discharge. Thus each menstruation signifies the failure of pregnancy to occur, the failure of a ripened and discharged ovum to secure fertilisation. But very soon after menstruation is over, the uterus provides itself with a new mucous membrane and the cycle begins afresh. A fortnight later another Graafian follicle has ripened, burst, discharged its ovum into the Fallopian tube, while the walls of the follicles form a new corpus luteum. The incretion of the corpus luteum stimulates the uterine mucous membrane once again to prepare itself for the reception of the fertilised ovum; and so on, da capo. If, however, on its way down the oviduct, the ovum encounters a spermatozoon and is fertilised, the monthly cycle is interrupted in a way presently to be described. In default of pregnancy, the menstrual cycle—consisting of ovulation, the discharge of a ripe ovum, the formation of the corpus luteum of menstruation, the proliferation of a new uterine mucous membrane ready to receive a fertilised ovum, death of the unfertilised ovum, atrophy of the corpus luteum, rejection of the disintegrated mucous membrane in the menstrual flux, reconstruction of the uterine mucous membrane, renewed ovulation—goes on month by month throughout the period of sexual maturity in every healthy woman. But there is another cyclical movement, life itself, superimposed upon this menstrual cycle. The child becomes a young woman, the young woman a wife, the wife a mother, and the mother a matron—this cycle being, as it were, a sort of extended counterpart of the ovario-menstrual cycle—the whole sexual life of the woman reflecting that of the reproductive cell, the ovum.

CHAPTER VI

General Considerations concerning Reproduction

Whereas in human beings reproduction is always effected by the conjugation of two cells, a male and a female reproductive element, there are many animals and plants in which reproduction is brought about in a very different way. Speaking generally we can distinguish between sexual and asexual reproduction, but there must be added a third or mixed type of reproduction which is occasionally seen.

Asexual Reproduction

The essence of asexual reproduction is that no conjugation precedes it, isolated organisms providing for the maintenance of the species. Substantially it is identical with the ordinary processes of growth, the only difference being that these do not lead to the enlargement of the individual concerned, but to the formation of new individuals of the same kind. We do not yet know why many living creatures tend to grow in this peculiar way by sprouting off new individuals and continuing their own life by the production of such offspring. It is, at any rate, an instructive fact that many animals (the tunicates, for instance) begin to reproduce themselves asexually before they have attained their full size. The growth processes leading to reproduction may either manifest themselves in a general enlargement of the animal, which then divides; or else in the enhanced growth of a particular region as a " bud " which, after a time, becomes constricted off from the " parent ", and forms a new and independent creature. This latter method is called reproduction by budding. In many animals, however, as in amœbæ and ciliated infusoria, a division into two equal halves occurs, each half becoming a new individual, so that it becomes impossible to speak of " parents " and " offspring ". In reproduction by budding, on the other hand, when bud after bud is thrown off by a parent organism, the distinction between parent and offspring is plain enough. Sometimes the buds, after being partially constricted at the base, remain attached to the parental organism, so that a family group is formed. The buds thus attached to the parent organism like grapes to a vine may themselves, in turn, bud; and such a process may go on—the buds in each case remaining connected with the parent—until an animal colony comprising many generations has come into being. That is the way in which sponges, many polyps, jelly-fish, and corals reproduce.

Sexual Reproduction

In sexual reproduction the productive cells of the female, known as ova, must be fertilised by the reproductive cells of the male organism, the spermatozoa, before a new organism can be produced. Such is the case, at least, when animals and plants are divided into separate sexes;

but there are hermaphrodite animals and plants in which the same individual produces both female and male reproductive elements. Parthenogenesis, or virgin procreation, may also occur in animals which at other times reproduce bisexually. In other species, parthenogenesis may be the exclusive method of reproduction. Parthenogenesis is characterised by the development of ova which do not need to be fertilised, but develop into new organisms owing to a spontaneous impulse towards this kind of growth. Often we encounter organisms in which parthenogenetic reproduction begins before the parent organism is fully grown. For instance, the larvæ of a good many flies reproduce themselves by parthenogenetic ova before entering the pupal stage. A special term is used to denote parthenogenetic reproduction effected by immature organisms. It is termed pædogenesis. In bees the worker females develop out of ova which the queen has fertilised with spermatozoa from the store of semen received by her in the nuptial flight, whereas the drones grow out of unfertilised ova. There are other animal organisms in which sexual and asexual reproduction alternate, one generation being produced sexually and the next asexually. This is known as the alternation of generations, and represents the "mixed" type of reproduction to which reference has already been made.

In all multicellular organisms which reproduce their kind sexually, the reproductive processes are fundamentally similar, and must here be briefly described. The reader will not, however, be able to understand the description without some preliminary knowledge of what is known as the cell theory.

The Cell Theory

Of essential importance to the growth of our knowledge of the finer processes that go on in living organisms was the demonstration that there is a fundamental unit of living structure known as the cell. In the eighteen-thirties the investigators Schwann and Schleiden founded the cell theory, which thirty years later was considerably improved by Max Schultze, and has been elaborated by a great number of biologists. In its generally accepted form the theory runs as follows. In monocellular organisms, those consisting of one cell only, the cell is of course an independent organism; but even in multicellular organisms, those consisting of numerous cells, the cell has a sort of independence, is a microcosm. Every cell originates by budding from a pre-existent cell or by the subdivision of such a cell. The cell is a tiny mass of protoplasm, a complex, semi-fluid albuminous substance; and every cell contains one or more nuclei. The word "cell" is rather puzzling to those who begin their microscopical studies with the examination of animal organisms, since the word calls up the idea of a box of some sort. It originated in the course of botanical study, for vegetable cells are separated from one another by a distinct cell-wall, so that under the microscope a thin section (slice) of plant tissue looks like a section of a honeycomb. The name cell for the fundamental elements of living organisms was conveniently transferred to animal organisms as well, although this honeycomb structure is peculiar to plants.

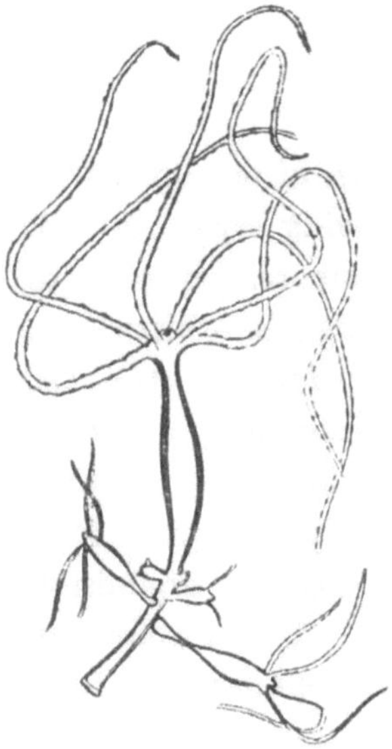

FIG. 22.—Fresh-Water Polyp in the Act of Budding

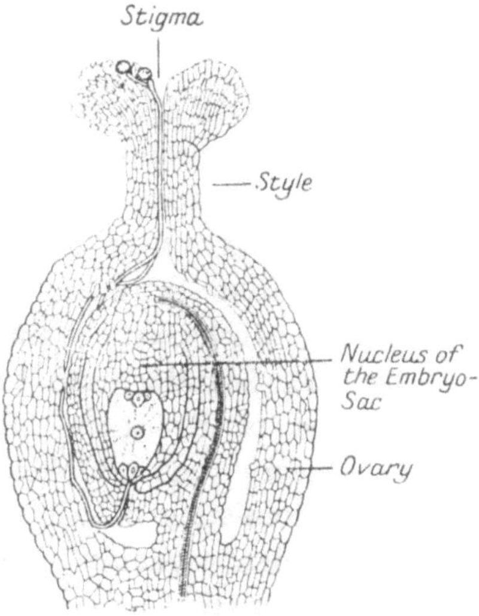

FIG. 23.—Fertilization of the Ovule of a Plant

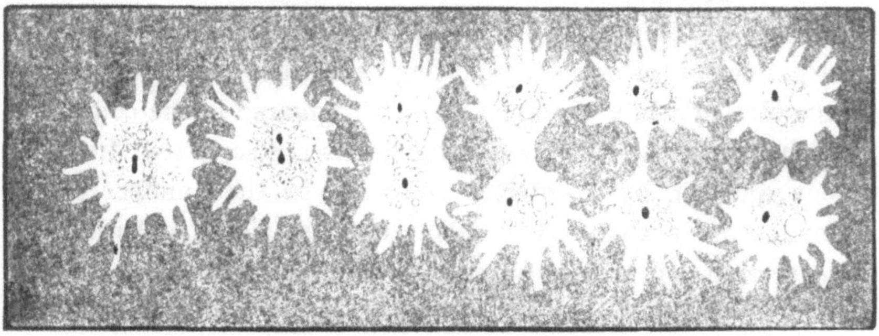

FIG. 24.—Division of an Amoeba

(From the Collection in the German Museum of Hygiene at Dresden)

Animal cells are for the most part small, but vary much in size, ranging from a diameter of three-thousandths of a millimetre in the case of the human spermatozoa to several inches in diameter, as in the yolk of an ostrich's egg. (The yolk of an egg is, before cell division begins, a single cell.) The typical form of an animal cell is spherical or ovoid; but through the effects of pressure, position, or other influences cells may become flat, prismatic, spindle-shaped, filiform (thread-like), or may throw out projections (processes) to become star-shaped. Most extraordinary forms can be assumed by mobile cells which proceed to absorb other bodies into their interior. As already indicated, some organisms consist of many cells, being termed multicellular, whereas others consist of only one cell, and are then said to be monocellular. A great many monocellular organisms are mobile, the movements being brought about either by a sort of crawling or flowing, thanks to the thrusting forth of "processes", or else, in the case of ciliated organisms, by the lashing movement of the cilia. As regards the reproductive cells, the female cells or ova of animals are motionless, whereas the male cells or spermatozoa are mobile. When in 1677 the early Dutch microscopist Leeuwenhoek first saw the spermatozoa of dogs and other animals (he had been anticipated in this discovery, though only by a few months, by Stephen Hamm) he regarded the rapidly moving little creatures as independent ciliated infusoria, and therefore gave them the name of "spermatozoa"—the little animals of the sperm. The characteristic animal cell is semi-fluid, its main substance being comprised of an emulsion of albuminous materials. The protoplasm contains, in addition, fat, carbohydrates, salts, and other chemical substances. The reader must not suppose, however, that we have as yet an intimate acquaintance with the chemistry of protoplasm. Since the fertilised ovum of a bitch can only grow into a dog, that of a sea-urchin into a sea-urchin, and that of a human being into a human being, we cannot but infer that, however closely alike they appear, and however closely identical their reaction to our crude chemical investigation, there must be enormous differences between the respective cells. Much still remains to be done in this field ; but of late years, with the closer study of the chromosomes (see below), we have begun to learn a little about the nature of the differences upon which the varying types of heredity depend. The main characteristics of protoplasm are its mobility, irritability, capacity for nutrition, and capacity for reproduction.

Conspicuous within the animal cell, especially when stained with certain dyes, is a sharply defined more or less spherical body known as the nucleus. Examination of stained cells under high powers of the microscope shows that the nucleus is shut off from the cell protoplasm by a membrane, and that in its interior, imbedded in the nuclear juice, is a sort of scaffolding which stains with difficulty. In addition the nucleus contains a substance known as chromatin, because it stains so deeply and so readily. For a long time it was generally supposed that the cell protoplasm was much more important than the nucleus, but in due course it became apparent that the nucleus controls the activities of the cell protoplasm, gives to each cell its specific character, and is the actual bearer of heredity. This can be shown by a very simple experiment, which can be performed under the microscope. If, for instance, we divide a monocellular animal, a protozoon, into a portion containing the nucleus and a portion devoid of the nucleus, the latter portion perishes very soon, whereas the part containing the nucleus goes on living, and can usually reconstruct the lost protoplasmic material. Cell division can be effected in either of two ways, one direct and the other indirect. In direct cell division, the cell and the nucleus simply become constricted and separate into two parts, the daughter cells, as occurs often in budding or in the asexual reproduction of the lowest kind of organisms. Indirect cell division is a more complicated process. It is presided over by a minute body called the centrosome, lying in the protoplasm close by the nucleus. The centrosome divides first, and then there appear in the nucleus contorted threads, which usually radiate from the divided centrosome. The process of indirect cell division is spoken of as karyokinesis, from two Greek words meaning " the commotion in the nucleus "; or karyomitosis, meaning " the thread formation in the nucleus ". Indirect cell division is said to be " mitotic ", and direct cell division " amitotic ". Mitotic cell division is only seen to perfection in cells which have a centrosome as well as a nucleus.

To come to minuter details, what happens in karyomitosis is that, immediately before division, the chromatin scaffolding of the nucleus forms an extremely convoluted thread, which becomes thicker and shorter, and ultimately breaks up into a number of separate rods, which are known as " chromosomes " (this means bodies which stain easily), and which vary in number from organism to organism. For each species of animals and plants the number is constant. In the cells of the human being there are twenty-four chromosomes. While this process of the formation of chromosomes is going on, the membrane enveloping the nucleus disappears, so that the nuclear content becomes continuous with the ordinary cell protoplasm.

Now the chromosomes range themselves in the equatorial plane of the cell, as regularly as soldiers in their ranks. Next each chromosome breaks longitudinally into two rods of identical size, and the rods of each pair thus formed, separate, ranging themselves in new groups at either pole of the cell. The result is that the number of chromosomes in the cell has doubled, there being at each pole as many chromosomes as were originally to be found in the mother cell. The fluid contents of the cell condense round the respective poles where the newly formed groups of chromosomes lie. The chromosomes at each pole join up end to end, forming a scaffolding with a centrosome, just like those that existed in the mother cell before karyomitosis began. Meanwhile, in the equatorial plane of the mother cell a constriction has appeared, a furrow which deepens until the mother cell has split into two halves, each half containing a nucleus of its own. The most important phase in the process of indirect cell division is the longitudinal splitting of each chromosome into two halves, so that thereby each daughter cell receives the same quantity of chromatin, which, according to modern views, is the real transmitter of hereditary character.

Such are the fundamental peculiarities of mitotic cell division both in animals and in plants. There are, of course, many variations; and it is a remarkable fact that in the

PLATE IX

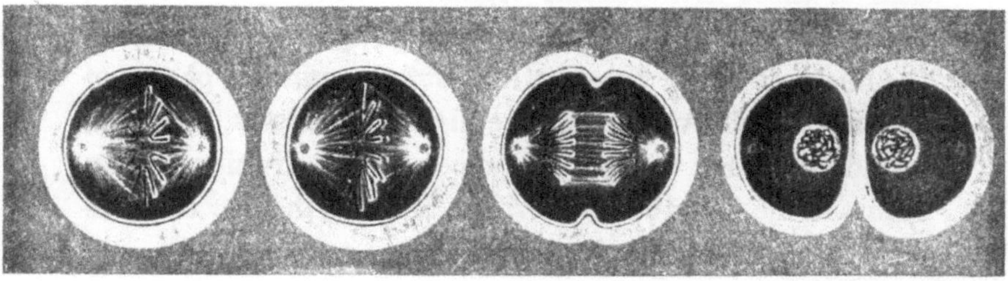

FIG. 25.—Division of the Ovum

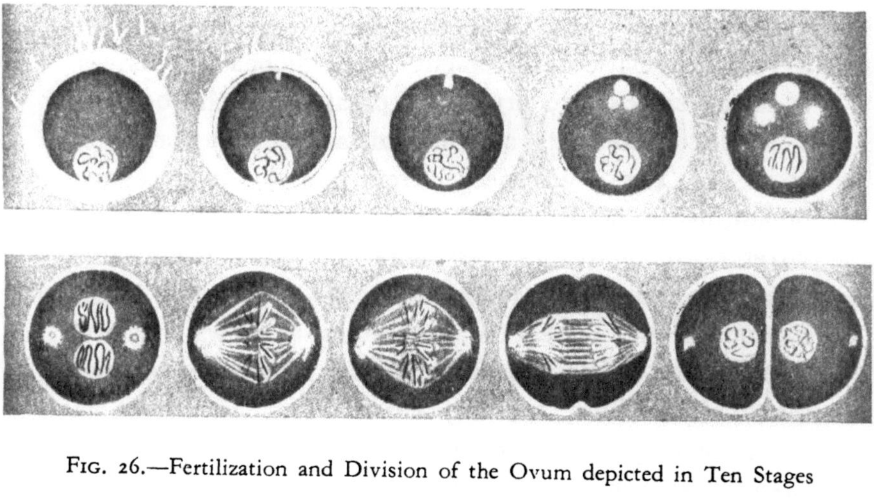

FIG. 26.—Fertilization and Division of the Ovum depicted in Ten Stages

(From the Collection in the German Museum of Hygiene at Dresden)

case of those monocellular organisms known as bacteria, whose multiplication can be very thoroughly studied under the microscope, we know little about the minuter phases of the process of division. In the higher organisms, however, including human beings, the process of cell division always occurs in the way above described, and it is thereby that the various bodily organs are formed during embryonic life, and enlarged during subsequent growth. An "organ", in the biological sense of the term, is a part of the body consisting of various tissues interconnected to form an anatomical and functional unity. A "tissue", again, consists of a number of cells of like kind. For example, the liver is an organ composed of various tissues; of the liver cells, connective-tissue cells, cells of the bloodvessels, and so on; and our description of the reproductive organs will have shown the reader that these, likewise, consist of various tissues. Thus as in the State, so in the body, we have a systematic development of cell unions into tissues, of tissue unions into organs, of organs into the body as a whole. Zoologists and botanists are accustomed to speak of the "advance" from simple monocellular organisms to multicellular organisms, and among these latter of an "advance" to more and more complicated organisms, ranging up to the mammals and to man in the foremost front of creation. According to views that still prevail, the entire animal kingdom constitutes a vast hierarchical edifice aspiring heavenward, an edifice in which each species represents a higher and better storey than the one beneath. Such a view found expression in what is known as Haeckel's biogenetic law: "The development of the individual, brought about by the working of the laws of inheritance and adaptation, is a condensed repetition of the development of the species; for, in technical language, ontogenesis is a recapitulation of phylogenesis—in a word, each individual, in the course of its development, passes through the phases through which the species to which it belongs has passed in the course of its evolution." To the present writers, such a hierarchical way of looking upon the animal and vegetable kingdom seems vitiated by anthropocentrism, the outcome of man's arrogant inclination to regard himself as the crown of creation. Nature, everlasting and infinitely great, knows nothing of human valuations. There is no warrant for the way in which we tend to speak of the division of an amœba into two equal and homogeneous parts as simple and uncomplicated, and of the production of a human being by the conjugation of an ovum and a spermatozoon and of the subsequent embryological processes as more complicated than the division of an amœba or as standing "higher" in the organic scale. All that we are entitled to say is that to our human understanding one process seems more complicated than the other.

CHAPTER VII

Fertilisation

The coalescence of ovum and spermatozoon takes place in the following way. In the act of intercourse, the semen, containing many millions of spermatozoa, is deposited in the posterior vaginal fornix. The number of spermatozoa in an ejaculation is almost incredibly large. Lode estimated it at round about 228 millions, but more recent investigations lead us to suppose that it is much greater than this. By such profusion nature has seen to it that at least one of the numberless spermatozoa shall overcome the various obstacles in the path, and shall attain the goal of fusion with the ovum. A considerable proportion of the spermatozoa enter the os uteri, the aperture in the cervix, thus finding their way into the cervical canal, whose mucous membrane is lined with ciliated epithelium—the cilia waving downwards towards the outlet. The ciliary movement thus retards the advance of the spermatozoa towards the ovum ; and when they enter the Fallopian tube they still have to swim against the stream. A spermatozoon is very lively in its movements, being capable of swimming as much as two or three millimetres in a minute. Since the total distance from the os uteri to the uterine aperture of the tubes is from 160 to 200 millimetres, a spermatozoon, traversing its own length in a second, could cover the whole distance in an hour or two. Probably, however, the ciliary movement above mentioned makes the upward movement slower than this. In a rabbit, spermatozoa have been found upon the fimbriæ of the Fallopian infundibulum two hours and three-quarters after coitus. In a woman who died during the act of intercourse, Birch-Hirschfeld discovered spermatozoa in the oviducts about fifteen hours after death.

The ovum has no power of independent movement, being passive as it is shot from the bursting Graafian follicle into the Fallopian tube and as it moves along this tube towards the uterus. Its reception by the tube usually occurs in the following way. The trumpet-shaped end of the Fallopian tube lies in a sort of pouch of the peritoneum (the lining membrane of the abdominal cavity), so that the open end of the trumpet faces the ovary. Thanks to this arrangement a " misfire ", an escape of the ovum into the abdominal cavity, is rare. The conjugation of the ovum with a spermatozoon usually takes place high up in the Fallopian tube. Thereafter the fertilised ovum is, in the course of the the next few days, swept down into the interior of the uterus by the ciliary movement within the Fallopian tube, and becomes imbedded in the uterine mucous membrane. We have no precise knowledge as to the time which usually elapses after coitus before fertilisation occurs, but there is a good deal of evidence to show that the time may be considerable—as long as a week or even a fortnight. Partly for this reason, because the exact date of fertilisation remains unknown to us, it is impossible to predict with mathematical accuracy when pregnancy will terminate. A forecast is usually made in the expectation that parturition (childbirth) will probably occur at the conclusion of ten menstrual periods from the day on which the last menstruation before the pregnancy began—the " period of gestation " being thus two hundred and eighty days, forty weeks, ten lunar months, or nine calendar months.

Having imbedded itself in the uterine mucous membrane, the fertilised ovum draws nutriment from its surroundings, the uterus itself enlarging concomitantly with the fruit it contains. Thus the walls of the uterus become very greatly thickened, and are far more richly supplied with blood than in the non-pregnant condition. In a word, changes take place in the womb to adapt this organ to its new functions.

CHAPTER VIII

Development of the Embryo

Others before Oskar Hertwig had watched the fusion of ovum and spermatozoon in various animals, but Hertwig's studies of this process in the transparent ovum of the sea-urchin have become classical. It was he who showed that the fertilisation of the ovum is always effected by a single spermatozoon. The German botanist Nathaniel Pringsheim was one of the pioneers in the study of the corresponding process in plants.

A prominence appears on the investing membrane of the ovum as the spermatozoon approaches, and it is there that the head of the spermatozoon penetrates, pushed onward by the vibratory movements of its tail. Directly the head has penetrated, a sort of coagulation sets in in the yolk of the ovum, leading to the formation of the yolk membrane which prevents the entrance of any other spermatozoon. The tail of the spermatozoon, having performed its function, breaks off and remains outside the ovum. The neck of the spermatozoon is transformed into a centrosome, while the head becomes what is known as the male pronucleus, the original nucleus of the ovum constituting the female pronucleus. The male pronucleus and the female pronucleus approach one another, and at length encounter and fuse into a fresh nucleus in the middle of the now fertilised ovum. Out of this nucleus arise the millions upon millions of nuclei in the cells of the developing embryo. There is every reason to suppose that the process of fertilisation in human beings closely resembles that observed by Hertwig in the sea-urchin. Here, likewise, there must be a fusion of a male pronucleus and a female pronucleus to form a fresh nucleus. In the cell division by which the spermatozoal element and the oval element of the nucleus were formed, a reducing process (meiosis, or reduction division) occurs, with the result that the number of chromosomes in each nucleus is reduced by half. Thus when the male pronucleus and the female pronucleus unite, the number of chromosomes in the new nucleus is one characteristic of the species concerned. "Unless such a reduction division occurred, two nuclei each containing the usual quantity of chromatin would come together, and the amount of chromatin in the fertilised ovum would be double that in the reproductive cells and the other cells of the parents. At each fresh occurrence of sexual reproduction the doubling would be repeated, until in the course of generations, the nuclear substance would soon become so bulky as to be utterly disproportional to the protoplasm of the cell, which would no longer have room in it for its nucleus" (Oskar Hertwig). We know to-day that the chromatin, the most important of the nuclear constituents in the female and male reproductive cells, is the bearer of those hereditary characters upon which individual peculiarities depend.

After the ovum has been fertilised and when its new nucleus has been formed as above described, it divides in the way characteristic of all animal cells. Its nucleus splits into two daughter nuclei, and then the process of cleavage is repeated and repeated, the number of cells increasing by geometrical progression to 2, 4, 8, 16, 32, 64, and so on, until after the twentieth division the number of cells will already exceed a million. Cells thus produced are known as blastomeres. To begin with they form a mulberry-like mass spoken of as a morula. This is a hollow sphere, whose coat consists of the aforesaid blastomeres, while its interior is filled with fluid. As it enlarges, the blastomeres, at first somewhat loosely connected, become more closely aggregated, and, forming as they do a layer of adjacent similar cells, constitute the first "tissue". Now the developing embryo has ceased to resemble a mulberry, and is therefore no longer called a morula, but a blastula or blastosphere. Its wall, consisting of the closely aggregated blastomeres, is known as the blastoderm. There are certain animals and plants in which the formation of such a blastula represents the adult phase of development. In all other animals (man included), however, by invagination of part of the wall of the blastula and the disappearance of the fluid that would otherwise separate the cells of the invaginated portion from the outer portion, the blastula becomes transformed into a little sac consisting of two layers of cells—like a glove-finger partially thrust into itself. This sac is called the gastrula. The layers of cells of which it is made up are called the outer and inner germinal layer. The "mouth" of this gastrula or "primitive gut" is called the "primitive mouth". Take a hollow rubber ball with a small hole in its wall and invaginate one half of it into the other half, thus squeezing out the air inside. The outer layer of the two-walled sac thus formed corresponds to the outer germinal layer and the inner wall to the inner germinal layer, while the aperture surrounded by the free end of the wall corresponds to the primitive mouth. This gastrula

Plate X.

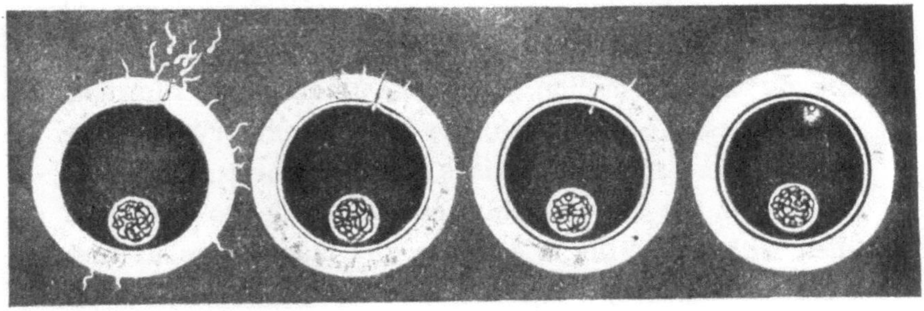

Fig. 27.—Fertilization of the Ovum

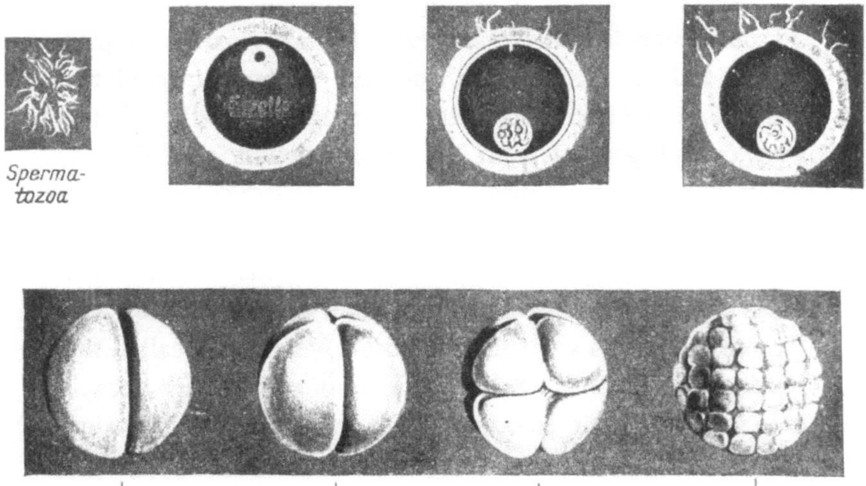

Fig. 28.—Fertilization and Division of the Ovum

(From the Collection in the German Museum of Hygiene at Dresden)

stage, once more, is the adult form of many animals, though it is but transitory in the embryological development of man and other mammals. It is upon these facts that Haeckel and his supporters founded their theory that individual development is a recapitulation of the development of the species.

Between these two cell-layers forming the gastrula, sometimes distinguished as the primary germinal layers, there now appears an intermediate germinal layer, consisting of cells derived from the inner layer. All the organs of the body subsequently formed grow out of these respective three layers. From the outermost germinal layer, known as the ectoderm, proceed the skin, the nails, the hair, the central nervous system, and the sense organs; from the innermost germinal layer, the endoderm, derive the intestinal canal and the vascular system; from the intermediate germinal layer, or mesoderm, are produced the bones, the muscles, the peripheral nerves, the reproductive glands, the abdominal cavity, etc.

As soon as the primitive organs of the embryo have begun to form, it sets to work pinching itself off from the germinal vesicle. A furrow appears round its body, and thereby is segregated a region of the germinal vesicle which serves later for the formation of the membrane and appendages of the developing embryo. Gradually the furrow becomes deeper and deeper, until at length the embryo is only connected with the remainder of the vesicle (henceforward called the yolk sac) by a stalk which becomes the navel-string or umbilical cord. On its abdominal side the embryo is gradually cut off from the yolk sac. Simultaneously two sacs grow up over its back:

an inner one, close to the embryo, known as the amnion; and an outer one, the false amnion. The amnion forms a cavity filled with fluid (the "waters") in which the developing child lies.

Before concluding this brief chapter on embryology, a few words must be said upon the physiology of pregnancy and childbirth. Anything but extreme brevity would lead us beyond the scope of the present work, and the married man who desires detailed knowledge on the matter may be referred to special works on the subject.

We have said that the fertilised ovum becomes imbedded in the uterine mucous membrane, which proliferates and grows over it. The whole of the uterine mucous membrane during pregnancy is called the decidua, this signifying that it is ready to be cast out at childbirth, the general lining of the pregnant uterus being the "decidua vera", and that part of it which immediately covers the developing embryo being the "decidua reflexa". The nutriment needed by the growing embryo is derived from the maternal body through the instrumentality of an organ known as the placenta, called in the vernacular the "afterbirth" because it is expelled from the uterus very soon after the child is born. It is formed by an intimate interlacement of the bloodvessels in one of the membranes surrounding the fœtus with the enlarged bloodvessels of the uterine mucous membrane. The fœtal circulation and the maternal circulation remain distinct, but products circulating in the maternal blood pass through the walls of the vessels into the fœtal blood and conversely. As the embryo grows, the uterus increases so greatly in size that by the end of pregnancy its cavity ranges from five thousand to seven thousand cubic centimetres. Naturally the enlarged organ encroaches upon the space normally allotted to other organs in the abdominal cavity, but this does not usually cause any serious disturbances to the organism. After the birth of the child, the uterus (by a process known as "involution") speedily returns to somewhere near its previous size, the abdominal wall contracts, and, in healthy women, the only permanent trace of an obvious nature left by a pregnancy is the existence of white lines shining through the skin of the abdomen and known as lineæ albicantes. These are the scar-like remnants of slight fissures that had been formed by the stretching of the subcutaneous fat. Certain anatomical changes are also left by pregnancy in the reproductive organs, but these cannot be described here.

About 280 days after the first day of the last menstruation, the fruit is ripe to be brought into the world. Its expulsion is effected by powerful contractions of the womb, accompanied by contractions of the abdominal muscles and the diaphragm. As a preliminary, however, the cervix uteri must relax, and be gradually stretched by the bag of the waters (pressing through it in consequence of the uterine contractions) until the aperture is large enough to allow the child's head to pass. Then follows the period of expulsion of the child, in which the head has to pass down through the pelvis and to enlarge the vulval outlet until it can secure an issue. The time spent in labour varies greatly, and is much shorter in women who have previously borne children. In those giving birth to a child for the first time (primiparæ) the full dilatation of the cervix usually occupies about twelve hours, and two hours more are required for the expulsion of the child. The contractions of the uterus during childbirth are extremely painful, and are spoken of as birthpangs. They are not continuous, but occur at intervals which grow shorter as the labour proceeds, when the birthpangs or labour pains become more intense, the efforts at expulsion more powerful.

As soon as the child has been born, the uterus contracts vigorously upon the placenta, which is detached from the inner surface of the organ, and is then expelled with the membranes as the "afterbirth". At first a considerable amount of blood flows from the torn vessels, but when the uterus contracts vigorously enough the bleeding soon ceases. In default of such contraction, the bleeding ("postpartum hæmorrhage") may be dangerous, and, unless skilled aid is promptly given, fatal. The involution of the uterus normally takes about two months, and for the first few weeks of this period a bloodstained discharge from the vagina continues, a discharge known as the lochia. Menstruation is not usually resumed until ten months after the birth of the child, provided that the mother gives suck to her infant. It will not occur, in most cases, until the lacteal secretion dries up. It does not follow, however, that ovulation may not occur during this period of "amenorrhœa" (absence of the menstrual flow). It is a popular belief that a nursing mother is spontaneously safeguarded against pregnancy, but this supposed safeguard cannot be relied on. A married couple, therefore, will do well to take precautions against the recurrence of pregnancy throughout the first ten months after the birth of a child. Women who undergo a rapid succession of pregnancies tend to age prematurely.

PLATE XI

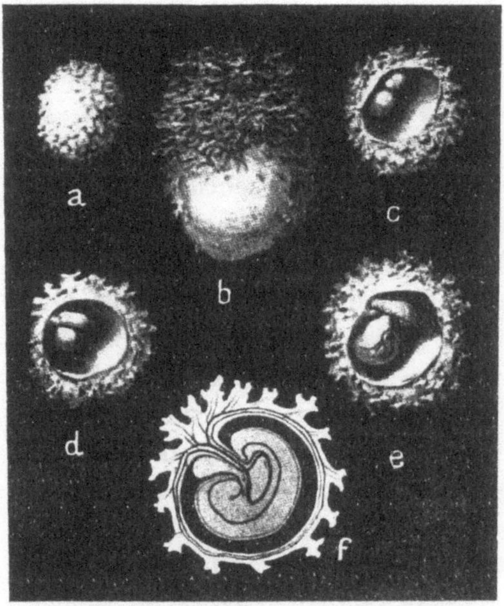

(*a*) Human Ovum at about the Third Week

(*b*) Human Ovum in the Tenth Week, when it has a length of Seven Centimetres

(*c*) Human Ovum opened to show Rudimentary Embryo

(*d*) Human Ovum opened, showing Embryo from above

(*e*) Human Ovum opened to show Embryo and Membranes

(*f*) Embryonic Circulation at Two Months

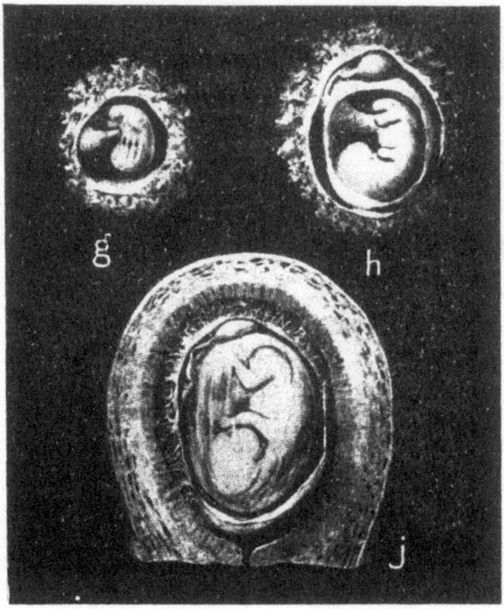

(*g*) Human Ovum at Four Weeks opened to show the Embryo

(*h*) Human Ovum at Six Weeks with both Membranes opened to show the Embryo

(*j*) Developing Ovum in the Uterus at ten weeks

FIGS. 29 AND 30.—Development of the Human Embryo

(From the Collection in the German Museum of Hygiene at Dresden)

What happens to the millions upon millions of spermatozoa which fail to fertilise an ovum? Many of them are simply expelled by the outflow of some of the semen from the vagina, either spontaneously, or as a result of the use of a douche. Though they can live a long time in the interior of the uterus and the Fallopian tubes, they perish speedily in the vagina, owing to the acid reaction in that canal. But even those which enter the uterus and the tubes, perish after a time, are broken up by the chemical activities of the female secretions, and the substances of which they consisted are absorbed into the female circulation. Van de Velde considers that these residues play an important part in the metabolism (processes of tissue change) of women enjoying the advantages of sexual intercourse. As to the spermatozoa which find their way all along the Fallopian tubes and enter the abdominal cavity, it would seem from experiments Höhne has made in the way of injecting semen into the abdominal cavities of animals, that these aberrant spermatozoa are dealt with by the body police, the white corpuscles, playing their usual rôle of phagocytes. Whilst the rule in the human species is to have only one child at a birth, in exceptional instances (about one act of birth in eighty) twins are born; and in very rare instances there may even be triplets or quadruplets. The tendency to produce twins appears to run in families, and to be transmitted by men as well as by women. Human twins are of two kinds. In some instances the twins have been derived from two distinct ova which happened to have been fertilised simultaneously and become imbedded side by side in the uterine mucous membrane. In other cases the twins are the product of a single ovum which has divided into two distinct embryos. The former are called di-oval twins and the latter mon-oval twins. Di-oval twins are much commoner than mon-oval. According to Bumm, the di-ovals form 85 per cent and the mon-ovals 15 per cent.

CHAPTER IX

Tubal Pregnancy

Should the fertilised ovum become arrested in the Fallopian tube before reaching the uterus, and should it succeed in imbedding itself in the wall of the tube and developing there, there results what is known as "tubal pregnancy". The arrest in the oviduct may be due to various causes. Sometimes there is an inborn deficiency of ciliated epithelium in the Fallopian tube, and obviously this lack is very likely to cause an arrest of the ovum. In other cases the Fallopian tube, as a result of infection (usually gonorrhœal), has been kinked, or partial adhesions form in its interior. Whatever the cause, the arrest of a fertilised ovum in the tube results in its becoming imbedded in a place which cannot, as does the interior of the uterus, provide scope and nutritive possibilities for full development. The consequence is that such a fertilised ovum will die in a few weeks, about six to eight weeks after the first day of the last menstruation. Then the woman, who has "missed a period", will notice a moderate discharge of brownish blood from the vagina. This will lead her to suspect that a miscarriage is imminent, and she will probably seek medical advice. Skilled medical examination will speedily show that the bleeding from the uterus is secondary to the death of an embryo which has been retained in one of the Fallopian tubes. Seldom, however, does a tubal pregnancy run so favourable a course.

More frequently the tube bursts under the pressure of the expanding embryo and something that resembles an abortion ensues, with the difference that the bleeding and the extrusion of the embryo occurs, not from the uterus into the outer world by way of the vagina, but from the Fallopian tube by way of a rupture into the abdominal cavity. If the torn vessels are small ones, there will be recurrent but not very profuse internal hæmorrhage, characterised by attacks of giddiness and faintness, by a swimming in the head, and by spasmodic pains in the lower part of the belly. If, as sometimes happens, an artery of considerable size is lacerated, the symptoms are fulminating. A woman who has hitherto seemed perfectly well, except that she has missed a period or two, will suddenly become affected with violent pain in the pelvis and in one or other side of the abdomen, will turn deadly white as if one of the large peripheral arteries had been severed, will have a cold sweat, and will very likely bleed to death within two or three hours unless an operation is promptly performed. The abdomen must be opened, the torn artery must be tied, and the blood that has been poured into the abdominal cavity must be removed. Even in cases of ruptured tubal pregnancy in which the symptoms appear less grave, the same operation is essential. In skilled hands it offers no serious difficulties, and a cure can practically be guaranteed if it is undertaken soon enough.

CHAPTER X

THE DIAGNOSIS OF PREGNANCY BY THE EXAMINATION OF THE URINE

THE prompt recognition of tubal pregnancy, even in those cases in which the symptoms of rupture of the tubes are at first comparatively mild, has been greatly facilitated by what is known as the Aschheim-Zondek diagnosis of pregnancy through an examination of the urine. Nor is this the only significance of this diagnostic method. It used to be very difficult to decide in many cases whether certain symptoms from which a woman suffered were simply due to pregnancy or were dependent upon the growth of a myoma (a muscular tumour in the uterus, formerly termed a fibroid) or upon the formation of an ovarian tumour—or, perhaps, upon pregnancy in conjunction with a tumour of one kind or the other. X-rays have, of course, helped us of late years, but apart from these it is no longer necessary to leave the diagnosis to time. The Aschheim-Zondek process of urinary examination for the diagnosis of early pregnancy has been one of the most important discoveries of modern medicine.

A good while ago, Abderhalden, the Halle physiologist, was able to show that the placenta is, in a sense, a foreign body in the maternal organism, for when fragments of placenta are introduced or spontaneously find their way into the maternal circulation, ferments appear in the blood which bring about their disintegration and disappearance. Or, rather, such ferments already exist in the blood of a pregnant woman, prepared to deal with fragments of placenta. If, therefore, the ferments in question are to be found in a woman's blood, we may infer that there is a placenta in her body, and that she must therefore be pregnant. For some years after Abderhalden's discovery, however, there was no trustworthy chemical technique for the detection of the ferments in question, and it was not until 1928 that Aschheim and Zondek were able to work out a reliable method, which is now in general use for the early diagnosis of pregnancy.

We have repeatedly insisted that the form, the growth, and the ripening of the reproductive organs are determined, or at any rate greatly influenced, by certain substances known as hormones, the internal secretions or incretions of various glands. As far as the female reproductive organs are concerned, the most important of such hormones is one produced by the ovaries. If, for instance, the ovaries of a white mouse be excised, the result of the absence of the ovarian hormone is that the animal no longer ruts. If, now, fragments of the ovary of another mouse be grafted beneath the skin of the animal whose ovaries have been removed, the usual phenomena of rut soon appear in the animal's vagina and uterus. Aschheim and Zondek discovered, however, that the ovarian hormone, when isolated, was not a competent regulator of the sexual life, inasmuch as the incretion of another gland had to co-operate. This other incretion, that of the anterior pituitary, is an essential contributory factor, serving, so to say, to start the ovarian motor. If anterior pituitary hormone be injected into an immature female white mouse (aged 3 or 4 weeks), the animal becomes sexually mature before the normal age, and passes into a condition of rut.

Aschheim and Zondek further discovered that in a pregnant woman, a very few days after the first period has been missed, the quantity of reproductive hormones in the blood is increased a thousandfold—so much increased that an excess is excreted by the kidneys and appears in the urine. Within five days after the missing of the first period we can, as a rule, demonstrate in the urine of a pregnant woman the presence of large quantities of anterior pituitary and ovarian hormones. Ovarian hormones, however, may appear in a woman's urine, under certain conditions, even when she is not pregnant. On the other hand, the presence of anterior pituitary hormones in a woman's urine indicates almost with certainty (98 per cent) that the person concerned is pregnant. Thus the discovery of this hormone in the urine makes us practically sure that a woman is pregnant, and the absence of the hormone justifies the conclusion that she is not pregnant.

Coming now to the practical application of this diagnostic method, it has first to be explained that the various hormones, if not identical in different mammals, are at any rate closely akin, so that, just as thyroid extract derived from a sheep can cure diseases resulting from thyroid deficiency in man, so the anterior pituitary hormone of a woman can induce rutting in a mouse. For the purposes of the test, several mice are used, since occasionally the injection proves fatal. The urine passed early in the morning by the woman suspected to be pregnant is injected into these mice hypodermically. Four days later the animals are killed, and their reproductive organs are carefully inspected under a lens. If the woman from whom the urine was derived is pregnant, we shall find, in all the female mice, that the vagina and uterus are considerably enlarged and are suffused with blood. Above all, however, in the ovary we shall note changes which can only be produced by the injection of anterior pituitary hormones. In those exceptional cases in which the appearances in the ovary as seen through an ordinary lens are not distinctive enough, microscopical examination will enable the investigator to decide with certainty whether the woman by whom the urine was secreted contained anterior pituitary hormone or not—whether, that is to say, she was or was not pregnant.

CHAPTER XI

Puberty

A CHILD is the offspring, not so much of those who are regarded as its parents, as of the species; and love plays its part in the forefront among the human instincts in order that the individual may proceed from the species. The sexual impulse or instinct serves for the preservation, not of the individual, but of the species; and it may become so powerful as to conflict with and conquer the individual's impulse towards self-preservation.

According to the researches of a number of recent investigators, and notably according to those of Goldschmidt, the sex of the individual is already determined at the time of conjugation of ovum with spermatozoon. The formation of the sexual characters is subsequently induced by the internal secretion of the reproductive glands. Beyond question boys and girls are strongly differentiated one from another in early childhood. It is not only the anatomical differences between the reproductive organs of the two which serve to distinguish a boy from a girl, for boys and girls have, respectively, a typical bodily structure, growth of hair, and timbre of voice; boys and girls differ much from one another when at play; while the familiar sex differences and many of the secondary sexual characters already exist in the germ in boys and in girls. The interests of the growing child are, so to say, sexually determined. A little girl is fond of playing with dolls, thus identifying herself with the mother, whereas a boy generally shows an inclination to play with soldiers and early manifests a puerile interest in elementary engineering and other details of technique. The boy is fond of imitating the notables of contemporary public life and those of history, whereas the girl extracts the material for her games and other amusements out of the incidents of everyday family life. It must be admitted that education and tradition may also play their part in introducing what are commonly regarded as "sexual" differentiations in these matters. Still, it is unquestionable that instinct is mainly decisive in causing the sexual differentiations of boy and girl behaviour. Even though the influences of sport are nowadays exerted with equal vigour upon boys and girls, upon young men and young women, the primary and natural differences between the sexes are nowise obliterated thereby. Still more do we find, when the days of childhood are over, that the sexual impulse and the awakening of adult sexuality run a very different course in youths and in maidens, being interconnected with the ripening processes in the reproductive organs, and above all in the reproductive glands, whose activity at this age produces such revolutionary changes in the bodies and the minds of boys and girls respectively.

Freud and his school, indeed, ascribe an important and differentiating significance to the sexual impulse even in early childhood. Düring opines, however, that the Freudians make the mistake of identifying sexuality (that is to say, sexual activity and sexual gratification as dependent upon the sexual impulse and the sexual functions) with sex as manifested by the conspicuous differences between the male and the female reproductive organs. At any rate, the sexual impulse does not normally awaken until puberty, the age when sexual maturity begins and the individual becomes competent for reproduction. In the present authors' view, the fact that many infants-in-arms masturbate does not suffice to prove that such masturbatory acts provide or can provide sexual gratification.

Shortly before puberty there sets in an enhanced activity of the thyroid, leading to an increase in the length of the extremities. During this period of growth in stature, there is usually, both in boys and in girls, a notable increase in weight. According to Baldwin, the most notable growth in stature occurs in girls between the ages of 9 and 13, and the most notable increase in weight when they are 12 or 13 years old; whereas in boys the corresponding phenomena occur between the ages of 12 and 15, and at the age of 14 or 15 respectively. As a mental accompaniment of such bodily changes, there is, as Charlotte Bühler has shown, a phase of enhanced consciousness of power, which is, however, transient, being succeeded (earlier in girls than in boys) by a negative phase whose main characteristic is a widespread failure of achievement, a universal bodily and mental awkwardness, the period being often spoken of, especially in girls, as the "awkward age". At the same time there is a marked inclination towards solitude. An interaction occurs between the thyroid and the other endocrine glands, which also become more active or sometimes less active at this period, the general upshot of such "team work" being the appearance of the "secondary sexual characters". Through specific changes in the bones, the osseous system of the young woman becomes more delicate, finer, and less angular than that of the young man—

a difference which persists throughout life. In the young woman the pelvis grows markedly wider than that of the male, giving the woman her wide hips and the somewhat "knock-kneed" appearance which is one of her most predominant sexual characteristics, though usually concealed in great measure by her dress. These changes in the pelvis are necessary to fit it for the act of childbirth.

A woman's legs, and especially her thighs, are somewhat shorter in relation to her stature than those of a man. A man's muscles are much more strongly developed, whereas he has a less marked development of subcutaneous fat, this applying, not only to the abdominal wall, the calves, and the breasts, but also to the arms and the forearms. That is why the woman's form is more gently rounded and more pleasing than that of the man. Another conspicuous sexual difference is to be found in the growth of the hair. In both sexes at puberty there occurs the characteristic growth of coarse, stiff hair in the armpits and in the pubic region, together with a vigorous growth of hair on the faces of men and an enhanced growth of the hair of the head in women. There is, moreover, a notable difference in the growth of the pubic hair in the two sexes, for in women this tuft of hair is of a definitely triangular shape, the base of the triangle being at the top of the mons veneris, whereas in men the hair tends to grow upwards, though somewhat more sparsely, as far as the navel. In many men, too, the front of the chest is hairy. Speaking generally, a woman's skin at puberty becomes more delicate in texture and better supplied with blood than a man's. There are also marked sexual differences in the voice. Whereas in children of both sexes the voice is soprano, in boys at puberty it "breaks", and thereafter in males it is tenor or bass, whereas the woman's voice usually remains high-pitched. These differences are accounted for by the fact that the larynx in women undergoes comparatively little change at puberty, whilst in men this organ undergoes considerable enlargement, as is manifested by its marked projection in the throat (Adam's apple). There are also differences in the type of breathing as between men and women. In men, except during violent exercise, abdominal breathing predominates, the air being drawn into and expelled from the lungs mainly by alternate contractions and relaxations of the diaphragm, whereas in woman the thorax expands markedly during inspiration and contracts during expiration. At puberty, too, the woman's breasts become fully developed, owing to an abundant local development of fat, so that the organs project from the front of the thorax and form a very obvious distinguishing characteristic between the female body and the male. In the male at puberty the testicles enlarge and hang lower than before, the left testicle being commonly at a somewhat lower level than the right. Erections have usually occurred from time to time in boys before puberty, but they now become much more frequent, and nocturnal emissions begin. In girls menstruation is established, although it is usually a little while before the periods become regular.

Simultaneously, as this process of bodily ripening goes on, there occurs an analogous revolution in the mentality, so that the neuter child begins to develop a masculine or a feminine personality. The mental changes and the bodily are, in truth, an interacting unity. It is now that the permanent character traits which constitute

" individuality " begin to find decisive expression. Often enough, children that have been bright, diligent, and docile, will, as puberty approaches, show themselves to be lazy, unstable, intractable. Conversely, in children that have been " difficult " and inapt to learn, there may often be noted at puberty a sudden awakening of interest in their studies, a marked improvement in attention and in memory. There are numerous transitional grades between these extremes, and sometimes what we note is a straightforward development of the aptitudes, inclinations, and characteristics that have already been manifested in childhood. In any case, puberty is a critical age, tasking to the utmost the capacity of parents and teachers, who often fail to realise how much care it behoves them to lavish upon children at this time of life. At puberty " young people " tend to discover a will of their own, to manifest a strong desire for independence, which may in pathological instances exhibit itself in the form of fugues (running away). Side by side with paroxysms of unruliness, contradictoriness, and fractiousness, there may occur a change of sentiment towards other members of the household or towards schoolmates and teachers, often accompanied by a marked change of attitude towards daily duties, and especially towards the obligations of school life. Tenderness, tact, and intelligence on the part of elders are preeminently necessary at this juncture. Firmness will no doubt be needed, but it must be inconspicuous, and exercised in such a way as to make the phase of transition as easy as possible for those who have not yet completely outgrown their childhood. Above all, parents have to understand that the time has come when their own selfish interests must recede into the background, since the fate, the happiness or unhappiness, of the developing youth or maiden will often depend throughout life upon wise or unwise management during these critical years of early sexual development. Grown-ups have got to realize that it is a mistake to lay much stress upon trifling manifestations of impudence or disobedience. It is part of the nature of the psychical transformation of puberty that boys and girls at this period are very apt to feel themselves unjustly treated; that they have a constitutional inclination to differ from their elders; and that they are exceedingly prone to make pert observations which they will be ready enough to deplore if the error of their ways is pointed out to them kindly and sympathetically.

Now is the time when it is right and proper for children to "break away" in great measure from their parents. It would seem to be an almost inevitable tragedy that young people at puberty should be misunderstood by their nearest and dearest. Nothing but shrewdness and sympathy on the part of the elders, enabling them to understand the working of young people's minds, can prevent the opening of a chasm between parents and children—a chasm that will hardly ever be bridged over. It is therefore incumbent upon the parents at this time to encourage their children's awakening interest in art, literature, philosophy, and science, thus providing a basis for fellowship between parents and offspring in later years, seeing that at puberty the child loses the sense of bodily communion with the father and the mother (especially the latter), the interweaving of egoistic and family interests being now severed. Only by judicious treatment of this kind can the parents minimise the risk of disastrous changes in character and avert the danger of serious disorders in their children's mental and bodily health. The task is a difficult one, for, strangely enough, whilst young people at puberty are very readily influenced by persons outside the home, they have a strong inclination to react against home influences, especially if these assume a dictatorial form. Parenthood is always a high moral charge, but at no time more so than when children are passing through the years of puberal development. Those who do not feel themselves equal to the occasion will do well to seek medical advice, which will often prove most helpful.

In both sexes, then, the period of psychosexual development known as puberty is marked by a vigorous revolution in the affective life—as already said, by a change of character in many cases—but always by the acquirement of a comparatively fixed character and by the development of individuality. Young men and young women, at this stage, are aware that something strange is happening to them; but its nature in many, perhaps in most, cases remains obscure to them, and they will not be enabled to understand it without skilled explanations imparted by loving adults. Often enough, however, light (of a sort) comes first from schoolmates or other persons of their own age, with results which may be disastrous unless the information, which is incorrect or is imparted from a wrong angle, be supplemented and amended by kindly elders.

The emotional life at this epoch is subject to marked vicissitudes. Just as the voice "breaks" in the boy, so in both lads and lasses there may be critical variations from moods of extreme joy to the depths of despair, and conversely. Riotous delight on apparently trifling occasions, an inclination to giggle at matters which to elders do not seem particularly humorous, extreme readiness to be mortified, proneness to weep, outbursts of anger—these are all manifestations of the remoulding of individuality and the transvaluation of values which goes on at puberty. Constantin Brunner has aptly compared the emotional state of the developing human being during the years of puberty with what modern psychiatrists speak of as cyclothymia. In its extreme and unquestionably morbid form, the cyclothymic temperament manifests itself as what is known as alternating or manic-depressive insanity (folie circulaire), in which periods of frenzied and usually joyful excitement alternate with periods of the profound mental depression known as melancholia. Cyclothymia, as ordinarily understood, is only a mild degree of this, in which periods of marked cheerfulness, usually associated with a rapid flow of thought, restlessness, and talkativeness, alternate with periods of taciturnity and unhappiness. Many persons are affected by this cyclothymic temperament throughout life without ever becoming actually insane; and a mild degree of cyclothymia is extremely common at puberty, although most people grow out of it to acquire a reasonable stability of temperament. The adult associates of young persons at puberty must be on the watch for cyclothymic manifestations, must understand them, and must treat them sympathetically.

Such mild cyclothymia at puberty does not transcend the limits of the healthy and the normal, but it must not be forgotten that there is a tendency for graver mental disorders to manifest themselves at this critical period of life, and sometimes to result in permanent insanity. When there is hereditary predisposition to mental disorder, both the years of sexual development (puberty) and the years of sexual involution (the climacteric) are dangerous to the integrity of the mind. Nay more, in this respect all periods when marked changes are going on in the reproductive organs are critical, so that in addition to the insanity of puberty or adolescence and the insanity of the climacteric, there is an insanity of pregnancy, an insanity that comes on immediately or soon after childbirth, and an insanity of old age—all more or less closely connected with changes in the reproductive organs. The internal secretions of these organs have, in fact, an exceptionally powerful influence upon the brain and mind of human beings. Still, it must not be forgotten that—according to the most recent views—in such cases the sexual hormones only pull the trigger, so to say. Hereditary predisposition is of primary importance in all cases of marked insanity.

Allied with the cyclothymic temperament are the facile enthusiasms apt to manifest themselves in young people during the years of puberty. In their inclination to admire and reverence some one, most often a person of the other sex, youths and maidens often select an object of the strangest sort, some person whom no one but the immature enthusiast would be likely to regard as worthy of idolisation. A girl at this stage of life will often conceive a profound veneration for some actor or actress, and will wait for hours outside the theatre in the hope of catching a glimpse of the object of adoration. The fashions of the day naturally play a considerable part in engendering such enthusiasms, and young men in particular are apt to be influenced by the image of "manliness" which happens to be current at the time.

Inasmuch as during this phase of sexual development young people are usually at a loss to understand the promptings of their own nature, it is not surprising that the object of worship will often be of the same sex as the adorer. Among girls, indeed, it is almost the rule that their first passion of the kind should be for some grown woman, often a schoolmistress. But in the case of youths likewise this is the period for entering into enthusiastic friendships which are expected to be lifelong. It is exceptional, in either sex, for the object of adoration to be the father or the mother, although an ecstatic worship of the father is by no means rare in young girls. A fact of fundamental importance in regard to these inclinations at puberty is that a great many young persons between the ages of 13 and 18 pass through a phase in which their awakening sexual impulse is not clearly directed towards persons of the opposite sex. Bisexual inclinations are, in fact, extremely common in youth. At one and the same time a lad or a lass may worship an individual of the same sex on the ideal plane, and be inspired with a physical longing for a person of the opposite sex and even enter into sexual relations with such a person. Not infrequently girls at puberty will kiss one another passionately or enter into even more intimate bodily relations while simultaneously carrying on an amour with a youth or with a grown man. During this period of bisexuality or of sexual undifferentiation, a homosexual adult may exercise such an influence upon the young bisexual person that the latter will acquire a long-lasting or permanent twist towards homosexuality, finding pleasure only in sexual relations with persons of his or her own sex. In the chapter on homosexuality, we shall emphasise our opinion that only in part do homosexuals owe their inclination towards members of the same sex to inborn peculiarities of their reproductive glands or their mental constitution. Enough to say here that environmental influences and seduction by older homosexuals may suffice at puberty to give the impulses a homosexual trend in young persons who, in other circumstances, would have developed normally in a heterosexual direction.

When the ripening of the reproductive organs has attained its climax, and when the bodily and mental accompaniments of this ripening process have led to the various manifestations of the years of puberty, there arrives the period (now sooner, now later, usually between the sixteenth and the eighteenth years of life) in which the sexually mature individual comes strongly to desire the gratification of the sexual impulse. For the present we shall concern ourselves only with the normal manifestations of that impulse.

CHAPTER XII

THE SEXUAL IMPULSE IN MALES

AFTER the transitional stage of obscure yearnings, the youth, now becoming fully adult, grows more and more plainly aware of his desire to gratify the sexual impulse. As a boy he was apt to despise the society of girls. Now he seeks the society of young women, and shows a preference for one or for several of those whom he encounters. What used to leave him cold as a boy, exercises a peculiar charm on him now that he is a young man. Indifference has given place to attraction. Sooner or later the youth becomes aware of the purpose of the external reproductive organs, and is seized with a wish to inspect and to handle the reproductive parts of a woman which, among civilized peoples, are concealed from sight by the clothing. If he has not been previously informed about these matters, the functions of the reproductive organs will usually be made plain to him in the dreams accompanying nocturnal emissions, which almost invariably occur from the time of puberty onward (between the thirteenth and the eighteenth year); and in many instances he will deliberately seek, by appropriate manipulation, to procure himself the pleasure with which he has already been made acquainted in dreams. In fact, if he has not been taught to masturbate, he will begin to masturbate spontaneously. By masturbation we understand the artificial manipulation of the genital organs until (in the male) ejaculation occurs. Another name for this self-induced gratification is " ipsation ", a term introduced by Magnus Hirschfeld. Masturbation or ipsation is practised by both sexes, and there are very few persons who have not masturbated in the days of puberty. The days are happily over when parents and teachers believed that masturbation works infinite harm to the lives of those who have practised it in youth. Physicians now see to it that the public shall become generally aware of the fact that most persons masturbate as a preliminary to the time when regular sexual intercourse begins. The injury to the nervous system supposed to result from masturbation is non-existent, and the idea that the practice can do permanent harm to the spinal cord is utterly nonsensical. Of course, excessive masturbation is harmful to the growing organism, induces nervous debility and excitability, and makes the person concerned less fit for ordinary activity. It is, however, hard to say where excess begins. In some young persons, and especially in young males, sexual development is unusually early, and may be accompanied by a premature and extremely strong manifestation of the sexual impulse. If these young persons cannot gratify their natural impulses in any other way than by frequent masturbation, we regard this, not indeed as desirable, but as the choice of a lesser evil when compared with premature indulgence in sexual intercourse—perhaps with prostitutes. A thoughtful conversation with the parents or with the family doctor; vigorous activities in other fields, taking the form of alternating mental and bodily work; the wise cultivation of intellectual interests, the practice of one or another form of sport; and suitable diet (especially as regards the evening meal)—will, as a rule, help to moderate the intensity of the sexual impulse and, if not to check masturbation altogether, to bring it to a considerable extent under control. Foolish parents who themselves make pleasure-seeking their main concern, who provide young people with unduly frequent opportunity for meetings and dances, and whose household is always in a whirl, can only expect that the result will be an undue erotic stimulation of their young folks and an accentuation of the tendency towards masturbation or premature sexual activity. In our own opinion, which is shared by the enormous majority of doctors, it is quite possible for a young man to abstain from sexual intercourse up to the age of twenty. Such abstinence does not involve any danger to health if the young man concerned has his life regulated in accordance with the principles above described.

The sexual impulse varies greatly in strength from one young man to another. It may be so intense as, in certain pathological instances, to induce persistent sexual excitement, known as satyriasis. Speaking generally, the capacity for sexual intercourse (potency) is at the highest between the ages of twenty and forty. There are, however, boys of no more than fourteen or fifteen years of age who have complete potency, and whose sexual impulse can scarcely be kept under control. Sometimes a vigorous sexual impulse and complete potency may develop in boys under fourteen, and in some of the Eastern races such an early development can certainly not be regarded as pathological. On the other hand, a comparatively late development of potency and a vigorous impulse, at the age of twenty or twenty-one, does not signify that there is anything wrong with the health or strength of the individual concerned. At about the fortieth year of life a decline in the sexual potency of the male commonly begins, and desire and capacity for sexual intercourse have usually disappeared completely before the age of seventy is reached—although in exceptional instances they may persist longer. The sexual impulse and potency are not necessarily correlated. There are men whose testicles contain active spermatozoa, although these men have never experienced sexual desire. On the other hand, there are men who can have good erections and can perform the sexual act, and yet fail to produce a normal ejaculation. In castrates, persons whose testicles have been removed, erection and a pseudo-ejaculation may occur, the secretion of the prostate taking the place of the true semen. This matter will be further considered in the chapter on sexual impotence. Even among normal men, potency is a variable factor, being dependent, not only upon the functioning of the reproductive glands, but also upon environment, mode of life, diet, and, above all, upon psychological relationships to the partner in the sexual act.

Albert Moll drew a valuable distinction when he analysed the sexual impulse into the contrectative impulse and the detumescent impulse, the former being the desire to caress and enter into close contact, and the latter being the desire to perform the specific actions which lead to the orgasm and the consequent disappearance of erection. Van de Velde prefers to speak of the " impulse to sexual approximation " rather than of the contrectative impulse; and what Moll calls the detumescent impulse he speaks of as the impulse towards the relief of sexual tension or as the impulse towards sexual gratification. In the sexually mature man the secretion of the semen and the distension of the vesiculæ seminales has so marked a reflex effect upon his whole emotional life that his desire for the act of union with a sexual partner becomes ever more urgent, until in the end it is irresistible, or can only be repressed by the expenditure of a vast amount of energy. All the same, we must repeat that the forcible repression of the sexual impulse is harmless to the male organism even during the years when sexual potency is most marked. Harmless but difficult! It is hardly possible, moreover, except in persons whose habits of life are sagely directed towards this end, and whose mind and body are kept very vigorously at work. Even though there may be quite a number of persons who live celibate lives without, for that reason, suffering in health, it remains undeniable that for a man in whom the sexual impulse reaches average intensity abstention from sexual intercourse must be regarded as artificial, and must in many ways restrict the full development of a virile personality. It would certainly be a good thing if to every young man who has reached the age of twenty possibilities were given for the adequate gratification of the contrectative impulse and the detumescent impulse—as happened among our own ancestors in more primitive times, and as still happens to-day among many savage and semi-civilised peoples. But the sociological and economic conditions under which we live to-day in western civilised countries make early marriage impossible for most men. Besides, it must be admitted that the results of the early marriages which were so common during the Great War and in the post-war period have not been altogether encouraging. To this matter we shall return. Civilised society has to adapt itself to the fact that, under extant economic conditions and in view of the impossibility of setting up house until a man has " got on in the world ", few young men find it possible to marry at one-and-twenty. We take a fairly optimistic view when we assume the age of twenty-eight or so to be the earliest at which most young men can afford to marry. What are the sexual possibilities during the seven or eight years that intervene ? There are three obvious ones : sexual abstinence (perfect chastity), masturbation, or recourse to the embraces of prostitutes. But there is a fourth possibility which will be considered by and by.

A good many men endowed with an exceptionally strong will, men of marked ability, men who are indubitably productive, manage to lead abstinent lives down to the end of their third decade without any impairment of their bodily and mental balance. But for the generality, this solution would seem to be impossible. As to masturbation, while, as we have said, it may be harmless during the years of puberty and very early manhood, its long-continued use as a substitute for sexual intercourse cannot but be regarded as injurious. Again and again we doctors find that masturbation practised far on into adult life has greatly reduced or even destroyed the capacity for normal sexual intercourse, and that men who have continued to masturbate until the end of the twenties are extremely apt to become affected with severe neurasthenia.

Having considered the alternatives of abstinence and masturbation, let us now turn to prostitution. The essential nature of, the justification for, and the significance of this institution will be considered in another connection. What we are concerned with at the moment is the question of recourse to prostitutes for the relief of sexual tension in bachelors between the ages of twenty and thirty. Prostitution used to play a very extensive part, and in many respects a disastrous one, in the preconjugal gratification of masculine sexual desire. It still plays an extensive part, though perhaps less extensive than of old. Men are more polygamous than women. The reader will please note that we say " more " polygamous—this implying that we differ from the view often expressed in works on the sexual life that, whereas men are polygamously, women are monogamously inclined. Enough for the moment to express our opinion that while women, too, have polygamous tendencies, these tendencies are much more strongly developed in men. As a result of this polygamous disposition of males, there arises a widespread demand for purchasable instruments of sexual gratification, whose individuality is of little or no moment provided that, physically considered, they are competent to minister to the urgent need. History shows that in all ages there has existed a class of women ready, in response to this demand, to supply their bodies to men for temporary use in return for a money payment or its equivalent. Such a meretricious relationship is, however, an unworthy one both for the male who hires and for the female who is hired. The dangers entailed by prostitution alike for the individual and for the community (because of its tendency to spread venereal diseases) need hardly be insisted on. In general, moreover, men are coarsened by regular intercourse with prostitutes. Besides, there is a close interconnection between prostitution and criminality, this involving persistent and serious sociological dangers. As regards the penultimate consideration, it cannot be denied that there are a good many men, tough-minded and not easily influenced for harm, to whom occasional preconjugal intercourse with prostitutes would seem to have been innocuous—but, even so, the risk of bodily infection with one or another venereal disorder remains. Taking it all in all, prostitution cannot be regarded as a satisfactory means for the gratification of the sexual need of young men during the years before marriage.

It would, of course, be utopian to look for the complete disappearance of prostitution in any land or in any future age. Even in Soviet Russia, the social revolution and restratification of the last few years has not resulted in the disappearance of prostitution, and has not even brought about a decline in the number of prostitutes. Prostitution, in fact, is a necessary evil, which will persist until an overwhelming majority of young men succeed in finding a corresponding number of women who will join with them in sexual relations able to provide a gratification in which mental love accompanies the act of conjugation—a gratification which therefore stands at a higher level than that of the immediate satisfaction of the contrectative and detumescent impulses. The sexual impulse, and the pleasure its gratification provides, are implanted by nature as a lure to the act of reproduction whereby the maintenance of the species is assured. Sometimes, therefore, writers on this topic speak of a " reproductive impulse " In the present writers' view, however, there is no such thing as a reproductive impulse, at any rate as far as men are concerned. It is true that in a mature man endowed with a strong sense of responsibility, love for his helpmate together with his own self-assertive impulse may, in the long run, arouse in him a desire to perpetuate himself in offspring, born of the woman he loves. At work here is the feeling (though often present only in the unconscious) that it is the joint production of a child which seals the love-partnership of the parents. But rarely, if ever, does there exist in the male a true "reproductive impulse" such as may and probably does play a part as a factor of the sexual impulse in many women.

Let us return to our question: "What is a man to do during the period of preconjugal sexual tension, supposing that complete abstinence is impossible to him, and that he rejects both masturbation and recourse to prostitutes on moral or æsthetic grounds?"

We come, then, to the fourth possibility—the "intimacy" or "liaison". These terms are used to describe a sexual partnership, uncontrolled by law, in which a man and a woman live in intimate sexual relationships for a shorter or longer period, which may extend to many years. The "intimates" do not necessarily set up house together; but whether they do or not, the "intimacy" tends in modern times to assume the characteristics of a pseudo-marriage; to describe it, the authorities are inclined to revive the term of "concubinage"; and by those who are in revolt against the institution of legal marriage it is often spoken of as a "free union". The persons who enter into one of these intimacies are, by hypothesis, impelled towards the union, not exclusively by the animal desire for immediate sexual gratification, but also by a psychological sympathy, varying in degree, but at any rate competent to give the love union peculiar characteristics. In the partners of many a " liaison " or " free union ", there is a real community of interests, whereby they are " wedded " for a long time, and perhaps for life, though not legally married. Without straining the term, successful intimacies can be spoken of as " free marriages " ; and where there is true bodily and mental harmony between the partners they are often enough more successful unions than those sanctioned by the Church or by law. But there is a less happy side to the picture, inasmuch as the majority of intimacies are apt to be severed, perhaps before very long, and usually by the somewhat brutal decision of the male partner. Furthermore, women who are known to have lived in such an intimacy with a man are less likely than others to find a serious suitor willing to enter into a legal union. The duplex code of sexual morality is here conspicuously at work. Few wives think the worse of their husbands because these have had experience of one or more intimacies before marriage ; but men, in general, are more fastidious about the women they propose to wed. Of late years, doubtless, there has been a change in moral standards, with the result that you will find plenty of men who do not take it amiss that the woman they propose to marry should have had a previous intimacy with another man—especially when they themselves are not immaculate in this respect.

Speaking generally, therefore, we may say that of all the ways for dealing with the vigorous sexual impulse of young men during the preconjugal period, an intimacy, regular intercourse with a beloved and loving sexual partner, is the happiest and the most moral. We must not, however, blink the fact that it is a dangerous moment when such an intimacy is dissolved, and that even to-day the dangers involved are considerably greater for the female partner than for the male. The risks to the woman, as regards her happiness and her security, will be less in proportion as she (and her sex in general) has acquired economic independence and has fully established her claim to equal rights with men in all departments of vital activity. But, above all, this fact must be borne in mind. It neither comports with a woman's dignity nor conforms to her natural inclinations that she should enter into an intimacy which is likely to be terminated by the man on account of some passing whim. A further important consideration is that the entering into an intimacy is much more the expression of a mere need for the gratification of the sexual impulse for the man than it is for the woman. As we shall have occasion to explain at greater length in the chapter on the sexual impulse in females, for the average woman the control of sexual desire is much easier and interferes far less with the development of individuality than it does in the average man. Our final conclusion, therefore, must be that, whilst for a man an intimacy certainly offers the best possible means of relieving his preconjugal sexual need, so that he stands to gain—there are considerable chances that the woman who enters into the intimacy may lose her all. She may lose everything which, in more fortunate circumstances, nature can offer her, namely, marriage, the joys of motherhood, and family happiness. We hold, therefore, that the ideal for which the future must work is one of early marriage, even though it has to be admitted that there are grave difficulties in the way of this becoming an ideal for the masses. If an early marriage is to be successful, the partners must have accordant individualities, their characters must be fairly mature, and they must both possess a reasonable amount of experience and knowledge, in conjunction with a capacity for making headway against the storms and difficulties they will certainly encounter in their way through life together. Be it remembered that when we speak of an "early marriage", we are using the term "marriage" in the widest possible significance, and are referring to a union entered into in the hope that it will be lasting and which does actually prove lasting—regardless of the fact whether it is sanctioned by law or the Church or is throughout regarded by the partners as a "free union" or an "intimacy"

The result of recent changes in social life has been that for practical purposes "sexual hunger" has ceased to be a serious trouble for the young men of all strata of society. Far more frequent than of old are opportunities for entering into transient sexual relationships, so that it is possible to avoid both the Scylla of masturbation and the Charybdis of prostitution. Nevertheless, the discrepancy between what is urgently desirable in sexual matters and what is possible, will continue to exist, for the reason that civilization puts man in many respects out of tune with nature, so that he is not, as are many of the lower animals, in a position to gratify his sexual impulse whenever it stirs within him. That is why love-conflicts, the disharmonies of the sexual life, continue to bulk so largely in belletristic literature.

CHAPTER XIII

THE SEXUAL IMPULSE IN FEMALES

As contrasted with the man, in the woman of normal sensibilities the sexual impulse is far less dependent upon active desires and a craving for the relief of sexual tension. On the other hand, sexual love is in woman far more than in man an expression of her entire individuality and an attribute of her mental equilibrium. That is why Byron wrote: "Man's love is of man's life a thing apart; 'tis woman's whole existence." These lines from *Don Juan* find an appropriate place in almost every treatise on matters connected with the sexual life.

The anatomical and physiological differences between the sexes afford an obvious explanation of the way in which the sexual stirrings of the awakening male, implanted in him for superindividual purposes, become so early and so plainly manifest to the persons concerned. Erection and nocturnal emission disclose to the youth the functional significance of his reproductive organs, whereas in the girl, menstruation notwithstanding, the copulative and reproductive purpose of her genital organs does not become obvious in default of specific instructions. Another thing that accounts for sexual differences in this respect is that a woman's rôle in the sexual life is primarily passive, primarily receptive; she gives her whole self, her whole body, and not merely her womb, to the nutrition and ripening of the fruit when intercourse has been followed by conception. Much more extensively and much more clearly than in the male is woman's sexual love pleasurably tinged by the reproductive impulse. We have already pointed out that it is exceptional in men for the urge towards sexual union to have as a conscious pleasurable component the feeling of a want to perpetuate himself in his offspring. In woman, on the other hand, or at any rate in the healthy and normal woman, part of the instinctive urge of sex is a longing to procreate in union with the beloved male; and it must not be supposed that the decline in the birthrate that arouses so much anxiety in many quarters is an indication that women in general have ceased to be inspired with a longing for motherhood. To emphasise, however, the point now mainly under discussion, it has to be recognised that women are far more often and to a far greater extent than men impelled towards sexual union, not by libido in the bodily sense, not by an urge towards detumescence and the gratification of sexual desire, but by psychical factors, and above all by sympathy. In a word, for women, far more than for men, what is termed love is an essential preliminary to the sexual act. A normal healthy woman cannot give herself at brief intervals to a number of men for the mere gratification of their sexual desires without a serious loss of self-respect. No doubt there are exceptions to this rule, but they are infrequent, and mostly concern women who have some psychopathic taint. Yet it is undeniable that numberless men, especially in youth, can seek and find purely animal gratification of the sexual impulse, and can do so again and again, without suffering any harm either bodily or mental —provided that they are lucky enough to escape venereal disease.

Nature has prescribed that, in the sport of love, man shall be the pursuer and woman the pursued, that man shall play an active and woman a passive part. When the first love ties are formed between a young man and a young woman who find themselves magnetically attracted each by the other, who are drawn together by impulses transcending their individual purposes, the desires of the young man are (in general) clearly directed towards the ultimate purpose of sexual union; whereas the young woman, in normal instances, though she is aware of a somewhat vague inclination towards bodily contact (the contrectative impulse), has but the most indefinite of inclinations to bring her reproductive organs into intimate contact with those of the beloved male for the performance of a joint sexual act. That is the explanation of the passive attitude natural to woman in the act of kind. The first sexual union is always painful to a woman, owing to the rupture of the hymen, whereas the male whose penis effects the rupture has an intense voluptuous sensation notwithstanding the pain suffered by his beloved partner. For a time, in most women, sexual libido remains potential, being only awakened to full activity, and only culminating in a voluptuous orgasm, after repeated experience of sexual intercourse. Nay more, this desirable awakening does not always occur. Throughout life, quite a number of women have no other gratification from the sexual act than that of giving pleasure to their sexual partner. Nor does this necessarily arouse in them any sense of loss or deficiency. Thousands and thousands of women who have no personal gratification in the sexual act become pregnant, give birth to children, and, often enough, regard themselves as happy wives. In the great majority of instances, however, and especially when the male partner is delicate in his advances and is genuinely affectionate, a woman who has regular experience of sexual intercourse will sooner or later begin to experience the orgasm ; but throughout life the gratification of her sexual impulse will be largely dependent upon sexual harmony with her partner, upon her own bodily disposition, and upon her general mode of life. (A lack of gratification in sexual intercourse often precedes the development of what is termed " nymphomania ", an insatiable craving for sexual intercourse.) In the normal woman, and above all in the normal maiden, the sexual impulse is subordinated to love on the mental plane, and, as already said, a woman's love life is far more than a man's directed towards the procreation of children. Of course, we shall be told that these views are out of date—that woman's opinions and trends and sensibilities in sexual matters have undergone great changes in recent years. It is indisputable that nowadays, in all social strata, there is a great increase in the number of girls and women who practise preconjugal and extra-conjugal sexual intercourse ; and that a change of sexual partners is almost as common among women as it was among young men in pre-war times. Is that a sign that the sexual customs of women have at length become frank and " natural ", or was the earlier condition " natural " and are we to regard the present one as a sign of degeneration ?

It would lead us beyond the scope of the present work were we to discuss in any detail the various reasons why women, or many of them, to-day claim the sexual freedom which used to be claimed by and mainly reserved for men. This demand notwithstanding, it remains a fact that (as Brunner well expounds the matter) in the general view the actual sexual differences between men and women, the anatomical and functional divergencies both bodily and mental, must still be taken into account. Thus people in general "continue to hold that a man who has 'sowed his wild oats' is, perhaps all the more for that, a suitable husband, whereas a charming and handsome young woman who has 'lived her own life' and has perhaps had one or two illegitimate children is not looked upon as a suitable wife." Although the present writers would not go so far as Brunner, who remorselessly stigmatises a woman living in polyandry as a harlot, and although they do not fail to recognise that there are many more men than there used to be who are willing to enter into enduring (nay, lifelong) love relationships with women of whose polyandric inclinations and practices they are well aware—nevertheless, it seems to us that such "liberality" of thought and conduct can only be the expression of decadent and morbid thought in circles whose members cannot exercise persistent influence upon the world at large without endangering the stability of our present social order and civilisation.

In truth we are not seriously afraid that anything of the kind will happen. Because of our attitude upon this matter many of our readers will, perhaps, regard us as reactionary pietists, even though we hold advanced views and incline towards the left as regards other problems of sexual hygiene. Let us explain, therefore, that we regard it as extremely unfortunate to entangle the movement for sexual reform with politics. The laws of nature can alone determine what needs reform and what is capable of reform in our sexual life. Now, the discovery and the understanding of these laws has nothing to do with politics but is a purely scientific matter. It only complicates the issue and discredits the campaign against falsehood, hypocrisy, and the double standard of morality when sexual reformers hoist political colours. It is true that nowadays those who have done yeoman's service in the fight against bigotry and on behalf of the sanation of the sexual life will often be found to declare that the happiness of mankind can only be achieved when women are accorded the same freedom as men in respect of frequent changes of sexual partners. We cannot agree with these extremists.

Let us quote Constantin Brunner once more. This author describes the free-love community which existed in Tahiti when the island was discovered. The women knew no restrains in their pursuit of sexual pleasure, gave free rein to their polygamous inclinations, and practised infanticide. Brunner has the "Tahitian" women of our own latitudes in mind when he addresses the false prophets among the sexual reformers as follows: "Certain restraints have to be imposed on love because it is necessarily subservient to marriage, the family, society, the State, and human life. Those who want to revolutionise love, those who demand that love shall be subservient to love alone and that women (being men's equals) can have equal freedom with men in matters of love, . . . desire to loosen all the bonds that hold life together and, in a word, to wallow in love. That is . . . a theory of wanton lechery"

CHAPTER XIV

The Sexual Impulse and Marriage

What line, then, must be recommended in this matter of the double standard? Compliance with nature and with the natural differences in the sexual impulse of the respective sexes. Men are more polygamous than women. They can indulge in sexual intercourse without the participation of the whole individuality. Women, on the other hand, are less polygamous than men. The average woman, whose natural destiny is to become wife and mother, has much less need for sexual variety than has the average man. In western civilised lands, however, the social order and the social situation are of such a kind that for innumerable persons early marriage followed by the speedy birth of children entails grinding poverty. People in love are incapable of judging whether the object of affection is likely to be suitable as a permanent associate. Young people, especially, must be warned against the danger of rashly entering into a marriage which will prematurely burden them with the care of children. On the other hand, alarmed at the fall in the birthrate and believing its existence threatened thereby, the State tries to safeguard itself by fulminating against the procurement of abortion—with the result that the practice goes on underground. The penalising of abortion completely fails to secure the desired effect, merely intensifying class contrasts and class hatred. The well-to-do [in Germany] can get abortion procured whenever they think fit, under conditions which practically deprive it of risk; whereas for the masses this resource is only available under conditions which often entail danger to life. Yet for the great majority of our population, to allow every pregnancy to go to term would result in home conditions threatening the welfare of the children and the happiness of the marriage. The obvious inference is that these risks must be averted by the suitable application of measures of birth-control.

Be it noted that we are referring to birth-control in conjugal life. We have no sympathy with the demand that the sexual distresses of our time and the crises in many marriages should be overcome by the unrestricted preconjugal practice of birth-control or (as far as married persons are concerned) by extraconjugal unions in which difficulties are avoided by the prevention of conception. Because men, being more polygamously inclined than women, have claimed for themselves the right to change their sexual partners whenever the fancy takes them and opportunity arises, it does not follow that a like freedom should be accorded to women who are less polygamously inclined and to whom nature has denied this right. They are not justified in compounding for their husbands' escapades by similar escapades of their own. We reiterate that nature makes it impossible, without grave consequences, for women to be as free in these matters as men—grave consequences for themselves, the family, and the State. All the same, we cannot see what harm it would do to men (with the exception of the few in whom the intensity of the sexual impulse borders on the pathological) were they to control their polygamous inclinations more than is customary. There would be nothing unnatural in such self-control, and the often quoted phrases " variatio delectat " and " toujours perdrix " are but specious excuses for self-indulgence. Besides, the days are happily over in which woman was regarded as nothing more than an object of sexual enjoyment for the male, to whom, for this purpose, one woman was as good as another. Recent economic and social changes have given to women as wide a field of activities as men. Woman is to-day universally regarded as man's equal and comrade, and she has good reason for feeling mortified if in sexual matters she is assigned a lower plane than man. For this reason the modern man equipped with a proper sense of responsibility has to choose between according to his wife the sexual freedom he is inclined to claim for himself, and (on the other hand) putting the bridle upon his own polygamous tendencies in order that he and his wife may join in aspiring towards the monogamic ideal.

If the latter view gain ground, if the dominant theory that man is necessarily polygamous be abandoned, the movement towards according to woman the sexual freedom which has hitherto been accorded to men will collapse. But the ideal of a true monogamy instead of the mere semblance of monogamy can only be realised if the married couple be saved from the economic and sexual miseries that result from the birth of more children than can be adequately cared for by the parents.

In many countries the State regards its existence as threatened by the fall in the birthrate, and therefore does its utmost to hinder birth-control. Not everywhere, however, are such views held. A movement on behalf of the State encouragement of birth-control gathers headway. Resolutions in favour of public instruction in birth-control have been brought before the British House of Lords. Even in Germany medical men are awakening to the necessities of the situation. They are beginning to see that individual happiness and the welfare of the community would be furthered if the masses, though less numerous, were more full of the joy of life; and that the existence of vast numbers of poverty-stricken and weakly individuals is a menace to the community. They are beginning to see that it would be absurd to sell five thousand tickets for a theatrical performance when the theatre can seat only two thousand persons; that it would be preposterous to ship two thousand passengers upon a steamer which has accommodation for only twelve hundred.

This is not the place for a detailed discussion of the sociological aspects of birth-control, and it will be enough to point out that the more populous nations have not always been those most successful in the competitions either of peace or of war. The Lacedæmonians killed all children that showed bodily or mental defects, and the population of Sparta was always less than that of Athens. When Frederick the Great gained his signal victories over his neighbours, the population of Prussia was much smaller than that of her enemies. Examples might be multiplied to show that quality rather than quantity is decisive in the struggle for power among groups and nations. Millions are spent year after year by the State in order to ensure that the feeble-minded shall live as long as possible; millions are spent in the fight against tuberculosis and other widespread diseases whose extension could be minimised by the State organisation of birth-control. The result of the wide application of these measures would be a great improvement in the quality of our population within a few generations. The dread of having too many children by which so many parents are now affected may be regarded as a sort of physiological safety valve. The individual wife, the particular couple, fail to realise that the endeavour to restrict births (often enough in cases where more children could be properly brought up) is part of a mass manifestation, is super-individual. Nations, like individuals, have lives of their own; and what from a narrow outlook many may be inclined to regard as morbid manifestations, are now, when contemplated from a broader outlook, recognised to be attempts at self-cure on the part of national organisms affected with disease.

As regards the happiness of the individual man and woman in conjugal life, let us insist once more that a knowledge of the methods of birth-control is essential to such happiness, whereas ignorance in these matters means that the family is overburdened with unwanted children while the wife's health suffers because pregnancies occur too often and follow one another at such short intervals, or because the overburdened mother has recourse to abortion which is often unskilfully procured. We regard it as essential that the laws penalising abortion should be modified. As now in force, they drive hundreds of thousands of pregnant women into the hands of quacks. It must also be pointed out that the need for having abortion procured could be obviated by the general diffusion of a knowledge of birth-control; and also that some of the methods of birth-control help to check the spread of venereal diseases. It is most unfortunate that in this country [Germany] we are not yet legally entitled to adopt Magnus Hirschfeld's recommendation, and, without risk of prosecution, to give plain demonstrations of the methods of birth-control. In England freedom has been won in these matters. Norman Haire, the well-known gynæcologist, was one of the first to open in London a clinic in which married women could be instructed in the use of means for the prevention of conception. (Haire's was, indeed, the first such clinic in which every woman was instructed by a qualified medical practitioner.)

The physical foundation of every satisfactory love relationship, whether temporary, or permanent and monogamic (the most desirable form whether for the individual or for society), is that the sexual life of the partners should be harmonious. This harmony is unattainable if either the man or the woman or both be afflicted by a dread of unwanted pregnancy. In view of the existing state of the laws in all modern civilized countries (Soviet Russia excepted), birth-control is obviously preferable to having recourse to the procurement of abortion after pregnancy has occurred—and is certainly much safer for the woman.

The physical harmony upon which a successful conjugal life depends will also be impaired when one partner or the other suffers from some condition which reduces or annuls the pleasure of the sexual act. We refer to sexual impotence in men and to frigidity in women.

CHAPTER XV

Sexual Impotence in Men

Impotentia cœundi

Technical experts distinguish between two kinds of impotence, impotentia cœundi, or incapacity for the act of intercourse, and impotentia generandi, or incapacity for the act of procreation (although the capacity for normal coitus is retained). When a layman speaks of " impotence " it is incapacity for intercourse to which he refers, and we shall content ourselves with a brief reference to incapacity for procreation at the close of the present chapter. For the moment we are concerned with impotence in the narrower sense, with incapacity for the normal act of intercourse.

The sexual potency of the male depends upon the cooperation of the central nervous system (the brain and the spinal cord) with the reproductive organs proper (the penis, the testicles, the prostate, and the seminal vesicles). Impotence may result from local disease of any one of these organs, from some affection which impairs their satisfactory cooperation, or from some yet more widespread disorder. In certain cases, without bodily disorder, impotence may arise from psychical causes. We then speak of " psychical impotence " in contradistinction to physical or somatic impotence.

As explained in an earlier chapter, within the limits of the normal, potency varies much, as between one man and another and in the same man at different times, in respect of the duration of erection, its strength, etc. If a decline in potency takes place at an age when such a decline is usual, the man concerned often regards his impotence as morbid, and will feel that it makes life unbearable. In respect of this senile decline, moreover, the variations in the age at which it begins are so marked that we cannot lay down any rule as to what is to be considered normal. Speaking generally it may perhaps be said that a marked decline in sexual potency before a man attains the age of fifty may be looked upon as morbid. When such a decline sets in after fifty, it must be left to the doctor in each case to decide whether the failure of power is normal or pathological.

No less difficult is it to state the "normal" frequency of the sexual act; to say that such or such a frequency is subnormal, normal, or supernormal. There are extensive individual differences in this matter, potency being, as already indicated, dependent upon the most multifarious factors. A man's occupation, the grade he has reached in the occupational hierarchy, the extent to which his work monopolises his energy, diet, climate, all play their part. Even more, however, is the inclination towards and the capacity for more or less frequent sexual intercourse a matter of personal constitution, and therefore these vary enormously from individual to individual. We can distinguish certain constitutional types which are characterised by more potency than are others. Constitution apart, circumstances have a considerable influence upon potency. Take, for instance, a man who, though still in his prime (say, about forty), marries a woman half his age. For the twenty years or more of his bachelor existence he has from time to time given free rein to his sexual desires, and has never learned the art of resisting the temptations of the moment. Such a man, when he marries a young wife will be apt during the honeymoon to be completely unrestrained in respect of sexual indulgence—and this will very frequently lead to premature impotence. One authority (Værting) has gone so far as to declare, that, as a counterpart to the movement for "motherhood protection", there ought to be a movement for "fatherhood protection" to safeguard husbands against premature impotence resulting from the sexual demands of their wives. We mention this as a curious point, without endorsing the recommendation, for we do not believe the danger to be widespread!

In town life, for persons who are actively occupied, intercourse twice a week may be regarded as an average frequency. Orlowski and a good many other authorities declare that during the years of utmost potency, say from the age of twenty-five to that of thirty-five, daily acts of intercourse (not more than once a day or night) cannot be considered injurious. The present authors are dubious as to the safety of such frequent indulgence. On the other hand they certainly agree with Orlowski that to have several acts of intercourse in one night is likely to prove harmful. Orlowski believes that a bachelor who, as is common enough, visits his inamorata or a prostitute once a week and then has repeated acts of intercourse may be expected to become impotent in the early forties. "Such a man has used up his potency, just as in childhood he lost his milk-teeth; and in other respects he may remain healthy and vigorous." If the view be sound, this type of impotence must be regarded as quasi-physiological, and the attempt to treat it medically would be futile. Nor must we regard as genuine impotence or as a morbid manifestation the incapacity of a man to have a satisfactory erection and to effect ejaculation in intercourse with one woman, when, with another partner, he is perfectly efficient in these respects. Such a condition of relative impotence has its counterpart in a good many women, who will be frigid and unresponsive in intercourse with one man, while they have plenty of libido and achieve orgasm in intercourse with another. We wish, however, to take this opportunity of insisting once more that the current talk about the polygamous disposition of the male as contrasted with the monogamous disposition of the female does not lead us to accept as valid the famous catchword " variatio delectat "—at any rate, to the extent of justifying a frequent or even an occasional change of sexual partners by men. (Still less do we approve of the way in which, in many circles, women have been inclined of late to claim equal rights in this respect.) Of course, it frequently happens that newly married men who for years before marriage have been accustomed to sexual relationships on a purely animal plane—to intercourse with women towards whom they were attracted by nothing but bodily need—prove impotent when they try to consummate marriage. Elderly roués, in particular, inspired for the first time with real affection, respect, and veneration for a woman, will often prove temporarily or permanently incapable of completing intercourse. In part the trouble depends upon the memory-traces left by oft-repeated acts of extra-conjugal intercourse, whose repetition in the changed conditions is felt, consciously or unconsciously, to be a sort of desecration. A "guilt complex" of this kind may make such a man permanently impotent vis-à-vis his wife, although he remains perfectly capable of performing the sexual act with prostitutes.

The profound significance of this psycho-physical mechanism has been admirably expounded by Freud, whose researches have done so much to make the matter comprehensible. We cannot here attempt a detailed discussion of the importance of psychoanalysis, whether in general, or as regards the analytical treatment of impotence and the sexual neuroses. We think that Freud's adherents and disciples have done a good deal to obscure the teachings of their master, but we have no thought of underestimating the importance of Freud's discoveries or of attempting to pass a final judgment upon psychoanalysis as a dynamic psychology. Still, we cannot but hold that a good many analysts overestimate the practical significance of their art, and tend to enlarge unduly the scope of their concept of the libido.

In Freud's view impotence, at any rate when it appears in a fairly young man, is always determined by psychical processes. The Freudian school holds that the sexual life of every human being finds expression in very early childhood in the form of the libido. This libido, which in the original meaning of the term denotes a craving for sexual gratification, is very variously defined both by Freud himself and by his pupils. In normal conditions, say the Freudians, the little boy has an unconscious sexual leaning towards his mother, and the little girl an unconscious sexual leaning towards her father. As an outcome of this heterosexual passion for one of the parents, a sense of rivalry results, leading the little boy to regard his father and the little girl to regard her mother with jealous hatred. These feelings are " repressed into the unconscious ". They are never fully realized in the conscious waking experiences of the children concerned, but they disclose themselves during sleep in a dream symbolism compounded of outcrops from the unconscious conjoined with memories of recent daily experiences. The heterosexual liaison with the parents, the sense of rivalry, and the longing to destroy the father or the mother as the case may be, repressed into the unconscious of the girl or the boy, is one of the many " complexes " described by the Freudians. This particular complex upon which the utmost importance is laid in their doctrine, they term the " Oedipus complex " in memory of the Greek myth of Oedipus who slew his father Laius and married his mother Jocasta.

The " repression " into the unconscious is, however, not always complete. From time to time the hidden feeling may peep out into consciousness, usually in a way which is unpleasant to or unfortunate for the person concerned. This is most likely to happen after the attainment of sexual maturity, with the result that the young man will feel sexually attracted towards women who in one way or another have an erotic kinship with the mother towards whom he was sexually allured in his childhood's days. Conversely a girl will be sexually attracted by men who recall the image of her father. On the other hand, according to the Freudian theory, the image of the greatly desired mother which has been present in the unconscious in conjunction with the incestuous yearnings natural to every human being (incest dreams, etc.), will often lead a man to choose as his sexual partner a woman whose type is definitely contrasted with that of his mother. Sometimes his unconscious or half-conscious revolt against incestuous longings develops late, and this, says Freud, explains why a man who to begin with had his sexual desires aroused by a woman of the same type as his mother, will subsequently, stirred by an unconscious sense of guilt, find that the incest wish of his youthful days is being symbolised in the act of copulation with the woman of his choice. As a result of this unconscious realisation and through the working of the sense of guilt, the "ego" will punish itself for its sins by afflicting itself with impotence. This is but one of the various ways in which the Freudians explain sexual impotence. All the explanations, however, involve a reference to the Oedipus complex, together with the interpretation of incestuous dreams, and the use of the numberless weapons that are stored in the Freudian conceptual arsenal. In the whole matter, dream symbolism and dream interpretation play a leading part. (For details see Freud's *Introductory Lectures on Psychoanalysis.*)

While it will be obvious, then, that the authors do not dispute for a moment that Freud's discoveries bear the stamp of genius, they have often seen occasion in practice to deplore the consequences of the wrong-headed way in which many of his disciples have worked out and applied his theories. This is not the place in which to attempt a fuller discussion of the matter. Beyond question sexual impotence is often purely psychogenic (caused by the workings of the mind); and in such instances psychoanalysis will frequently effect a cure. Still, when cure results, it must not be forgotten that this may be the outcome of the psychotherapeutic powers of persons who are able to exercise a suggestive influence even though the doctrine on which their analytic method be based is false. In a word, the undeniable practical successes of many psychoanalysts can, in our view, be often enough secured by the application of other psychotherapeutic methods.

When sexual impotence is due to purely physical causes, this does not necessarily mean that the testicles or the penis will be found abnormally large or abnormally small. Again and again specialists are consulted by young men who are alarmed because the penis or the testicles are very small, and who therefore dread that they will soon become impotent. In not a few such persons transient impotence may be brought about by this very dread. Let us, therefore, declare most emphatically that a man with exceptionally large testicles or penis may be impotent, and that one with very small genital organs may have a marked excess of functional capacity. There are, of course, cases in which phimosis (tightness of the foreskin which cannot be retracted from the glans) or stricture of the urinary meatus (the external aperture of the urethra) may indirectly lead to impotence in persons in whom the conditions make the movements requisite for copulation painful. A minor surgical operation will, in such persons, suffice to cure impotence thus caused. In this connection we must refer once more to inflammatory induration, usually on one side, but sometimes on both sides, of the shaft of the penis, interfering with the proper filling of the corpora cavernosa, so that when erection takes place the organ is bent to one side (chordee). Local treatment is requisite for these patients, the trouble in many instances being relieved by radium emanations or by X-rays.

The most important varieties of impotence may be classified as follows: (1) Cases in which, though the capacity for erection and ejaculation persist, there is no adequate desire for sexual intercourse. (2) Cases in which the power for erection is lacking. (3) Cases in which the capacity for ejaculation is lacking. (4) Cases in which erection occurs satisfactorily, but, when intercourse is attempted, ejaculation occurs prematurely, often at the first endeavour to penetrate, and usually before the climax of sexual pleasure is reached.

(1) The lack of adequate longing for the performance of the copulatory act, insufficient libido, seldom exists for any considerable time without the capacity for erection becoming more and more impaired. All the more will this arise when the situation is complicated by the failure of the orgasm to be sufficiently pleasurable, or when ejaculation is actually painful. As a cause of unsufficiency of libido there will usually be found to exist a general condition of neurasthenic exhaustion, especially as a sequel of certain infectious disorders, such as influenza, typhoid, scarlatina, etc. Poisoning with quinine, lead, and other chemical substances is sometimes responsible for the trouble. The prolonged abuse of alcohol can also lead to a decline in libido; and so, likewise, though this is not so generally known, can the long-continued abuse of tobacco. Business cares, anxieties, and excitement; insufficient diet; unsuitable climate—all of these may play their part. Physical examination of the genital organs seldom discloses anything relevant in these patients. Each case must be

treated on its merits, the most important measures being general and dietetic, in conjunction with the relief of mental tension, change of air, a separation from the habitual sexual partner, and the avoidance of any attempt at sexual activity unless the desire for it spontaneously arises. Sooner or later such measures will usually bring about a cure.

(2) When a phase in which libido is diminished or absent is followed by a phase in which erection becomes inadequate and in which ejaculation is delayed or premature, we often, though by no means invariably, find that there is hypertrophy of the little prominence in the posterior urethra known as the verumontanum or colliculus seminalis (described in Chapter II). In such cases treatment by a specialist will be required, and also when the symptoms are dependent upon some other local lesion, such as scars in the urethral mucous membrane as a sequel of gonorrhœa or injury.

(3) and (4) Failure of ejaculation, and still more ejaculatio præcox, is likely to be due to a general congestive and inflammatory condition of the posterior urethra, or to an irritable condition of the ejaculation centre in the spinal cord, or to both combined. Very often the long-continued practice of coitus interruptus will be found to have been the cause of these troubles. When, during the act of intercourse, the penis is withdrawn by the male partner immediately before ejaculation, the full relief of tension characteristic of healthy detumescence fails to occur in his genital organs, with the result that, in the course of time, the effects of persistent congestion are likely to manifest themselves in the posterior urethra and in the colliculus seminalis. It cannot be too often repeated that

the frequent practice of coitus interruptus can hardly fail to be injurious, and not to the male partner alone. Nervous disturbances of the heart in both partners are common results.

In other cases the cause of ejaculatio præcox, painful erections, or complete impotence is inflammation of the prostate, usually accompanied with slight hypertrophy of the colliculus seminalis. Diseases of the vesiculæ seminales are also occasional causes of disorders of potency. The underlying trouble is generally a chronic inflammation of these little sacs, the sequel of an extension of gonorrhœal or non-gonorrhœal inflammation from the urethra. Spermatorrhœa (the discharge of semen apart from sexual excitement) is often dependent upon such inflammation of the seminal vesicles. Even in healthy individuals the pressure of the fæces upon the base of the bladder during the evacuation of the bowels will sometimes cause spermatorrhœa. A man thus affected is apt to be greatly alarmed by the symptom, which, by its reaction upon his mind, will often give rise to secondary disorders of potency for which there is no sufficient anatomical cause. Of course, such mechanically induced spermatorrhœa during defæcation is more likely to arise when the seminal vesicles are inflamed and enlarged; but, unless the inflammation is tubercular, this trouble is not per se dangerous. Indirectly, however, it is apt to give rise to a good deal of trouble, especially in persons with a congenitally neuropathic predisposition, in whom the alarm the spermatorrhœa occasions is apt to cause neurasthenia. Skilled treatment will often relieve the patient's fear and thus cure the neurasthenia, but sometimes the mental balance is so seriously upset that the resulting impotence proves incurable. It must be remembered, in this connection, that quacks with nostrums to sell are wont to play upon the fears which spermatorrhœa and ejaculatio præcox arouse! The "specifics" usually recommended contain yohimbin, lecithin combined with phosphorus, arsenic, nux vomica, etc. In earlier days cantharides (an oleaginous or alcoholic extract of the Spanish fly) was a great deal used for the treatment of impotence. This is an extremely dangerous drug, for in many persons, even in minute doses, it causes severe inflammation of the kidneys. As regards all these remedies for impotence, classed together as "aphrodisiacs", we know to-day that their occasional successes are mainly if not exclusively dependent upon the working of suggestion or autosuggestion. There is, in fact, no such thing as a trustworthy aphrodisiac drug. Apart from suggestion, the restoration of potency that sometimes follows the administration of aphrodisiacs is often a mere coincidence.

Disorders of potency are so multifarious in their nature that in any particular instance, even though the cause will be obvious enough to an expert, it will be exceedingly difficult for a layman to recognise unaided what is wrong with the technique of his sexual intercourse and to modify his practices in such a way as to bring about the restoration of normal potency. It is of the utmost importance, therefore, that men who suffer or believe themselves to suffer from impotence should not waste their time and their money in running from one quack to another, but should promptly seek the advice of a skilled physician. Nowadays there is really no ground for being afraid that a specialist will be too ready to have recourse to the whole armamentarium of urology—will needlessly plague the patient by the use of sounds, bougies, electrical apparatus, and so on. Doctors of the present generation know so much about the mental substratum of bodily disorders that they are unlikely to make the mistake of showing themselves too active in the matter of local treatment and therefore perhaps making their patient worse. Besides considering the local situation, every properly trained physician skilled in the treatment of such disorders will, quite apart from a review of the local situation, look for more general bodily and mental causes of a disturbance of potency—for diabetes perhaps, for a syphilitic or other disorder of the nervous system, for some unfavourable factor in the environment, for some error in diet, in the technique of sexual intercourse, etc. Not until he has excluded such general causes, and not until he has tried the effect of general treatment by diet and drugs and psychotherapeutics, will he proceed (should these measures fail) to consider the advisability of instrumental examination of the urethra and of local treatment. In some such cases, perhaps, diathermy of the prostate and testicles may have a remarkably good effect, but this matter cannot be considered in detail here.

As far as concerns the general principles of the prevention and treatment of disorders of the sexual functions, deficient libido, and its consequences, the following simple rules of life may be prescribed. Obedience to the maxim "early to bed and early to rise" is desirable; and a reasonably invigorating mixed diet is helpful to the maintenance of sexual potency. On the other hand, late and irregular hours, disorderly habits, much rushing to and fro, and attempts to stimulate sexual desire by the use of alcohol, are unquestionably harmful. Nor should any reliance be placed upon certain articles of food and drink which are popularly regarded as aphrodisiacs, such as red wine, celery, strongly seasoned food, and so on. Their effect is extremely problematical, as compared with that of a reasonable and natural mode of life. We may repeat, in this connection, that the abuse of tobacco is as harmful to potency as the abuse of alcohol.

Very important in the causation of disturbances of sexual potency is an improper technique in coitus, taking the form of an attempt on the part of the male to prolong the act unduly, deferring its culmination in orgasm and ejaculation for as long as possible and perhaps indefinitely. Technically this process is known as coitus reservatus. When, with a view to the prolongation of sexual pleasure, the male partner "reserves" the orgasm so long that the erectile mechanism becomes exhausted and erection passes off before ejaculation has taken place, the practice is occasionally termed "Oneida", for such (in addition to complex or communal marriage) was the technique of sexual intercourse among the "Bible Communists" of the Oneida Community in the United States during the 'fifties, 'sixties, and 'seventies of the nineteenth century. This extreme form of coitus reservatus is sometimes spoken of as "carezza". In either form, coitus reservatus must be most emphatically condemned, for it is no less likely than coitus interruptus to induce posterior urethral congestion, hypertrophy of the colliculus seminalis, and grave impairment of sexual potency. Doctors in general do well when they utter the most emphatic warnings against the practice of coitus reservatus.

Van de Velde is an exception here. In his widely read book *Ideal Marriage*, this author, although he condemns coitus reservatus pushed to the degree of avoiding the orgasm altogether, advises the occasional prolongation of the sexual act, considering this advantageous to the female partner, who is otherwise unlikely to achieve adequate gratification. He also describes, with an unnecessary wealth of detail, " love play " as a desirable preliminary to the sexual act, in order to intensify the woman's libido. The present authors differ from him strongly. The " love play " thus advocated and the undue prolongation of the act of intercourse, may further sexual pleasure in women, but cannot fail to make a great many sexual neurasthenics among men. Above all do we strongly disapprove of Van de Velde's recommendation that immediately after complete intercourse the male should, if he has inclination and potency, start afresh on a new love play, communion, and orgasm. This will in general do less harm to the woman than to the man ; but the normal thing for both partners, especially for a married couple, certainly is that the sexual act should not be repeated after a very brief interval. A great many men derive the impression that they must be inadequately potent when they hear other men boast of a capacity to repeat the act of intercourse several times, perhaps six times or more, in quick succession. In most cases, such " prowess " is entirely fictitious, but the boasters would do no harm by thus gratifying their vanity were it not that they may make some of their hearers doubt their own potency. Nowadays, when such extensive and exhausting calls are made upon nervous and bodily energy, there is grave danger that the false prophets who abound on all sides may, with their erroneous doctrines about the way to ensure the happiness of married life, provide innumerable recruits for the great army of neurasthenics and greatly increase the number of persons affected with a purely psychical impotence. Greater caution should be exercised in accepting the advice of authors whose works doubtless bear witness to the remarkable potency of the writers, but whose advice cannot but be harmful to many of the readers who swallow it so credulously. We consider that the consequences of such unwise guidance are already manifest in the increase of psychical impotence. It would be far better to advise the men of to-day, already inclined to be neurasthenic, over-stimulated, and injuriously affected by the intensity of the economic struggle, to enjoy sexual intercourse in normal fashion, without extensive preliminaries, and without any attempt at artificial prolongation, but proceeding as quickly as may be to orgasm and ejaculation. In this way the wholesale production of psychical impotence would be avoided.

A good many cases of psychical impotence depend, not upon dread of venereal infection or upon distaste for intercourse with prostitutes, but simply upon the fact that upon one occasion the patient has failed to effect coitus, and has ever since been paralysed by the autosuggestion of permanent impotence. Whenever he makes a fresh attempt, instead of marching straight to his goal, he can think of nothing but the certainty that he will fail. Again, in men who have masturbated for years, the fear that the practice has injured their virility may cause psychical impotence. One for whom ipsation has become a regular substitute for the normal sexual act may thus be subject to a sort of feminophobia. Often enough, life will itself effect a cure, by bringing the sufferer into sexual relations with a bodily adequate and sympathetic partner towards whom he feels an attraction strong enough to overcome his phobia. In default of this, such persons can almost always be helped by psychotherapy, although the course of treatment may have to be a long one. In some instances psychoanalysis is more successful than any other method, but in the present writers' view the analyst's personality is of supreme importance in these cases also.

Lastly we have to consider the treatment of senile impotence. Normally, indeed, this is not a "malady" requiring "treatment" at all, for a man who has grown grey in work and in honour should resign himself to the fact that his potency must decline with advancing years, and that this decline occurs earlier in some men than in others. We regard it as preposterous that a man should wish or should attempt, by artificial means, to arrest or to reverse the process of growing old, which is the natural wearing out of the human body. Such endeavours must be classed with Paracelsus' desire to create the homunculus, or with the wish to square the circle. Still, in those who, through heredity or illness, become affected by a markedly premature "senile impotence", the method of Steinach or that of Voronoff may be tried. Steinach found that by ligaturing the vasa deferentia of ageing guineapigs and rats a restoration of the loss of sexual potency could be induced in these animals, the "rejuvenation" being dependent upon a marked proliferation of the interstitial tissue of the testicles (termed by Steinach the "puberty gland") and the consequent pouring of testicular hormone into the blood. The incretion of the puberty gland stimulates the other endocrine glands, reactivates the secondary sexual characters, and rejuvenates the individual thus operated on. The corresponding operation in human beings would appear to have produced temporary rejuvenation, but the effects were transient, and were in part unquestionably determined by psychical influences. Voronoff grafted the testicles of apes (chimpanzees) into ageing men, and claimed that in his patients the internal secretion from the grafts compensated for the previous lack of testicular hormone and brought about rejuvenation. Voronoff's experiments were repeated by numerous other surgeons, who failed, however, to obtain the results described by the originator of testicular grafting. They found that the ingrafted testicles, belonging as they did to another species of animal, speedily underwent atrophy in the human host, the testicular tissue being replaced by ordinary fatty tissue. The transiently successful results observed in a good many men can be sufficiently explained by the suggestive effect of the operation (the patient's mind having been prepared by the reading of sensational newspaper articles !). Still, it cannot be denied that the ingrafted gland may exert a fugitive influence, so as long as it still remains functional.[1]

If, however, there be no trustworthy cure for physiological senile impotence, there is certainly an excellent means of

[1] A much more sanguine view of "reactivation" by vasoligature, testicular grafts, etc.—a view based upon the reports of very numerous cases—in human beings will be found in Peter Schmidt's *The Conquest of Old Age*, Routledge, London, 1931.—TRANSLATORS' NOTE.

prevention, namely the regular practice of normal sexual intercourse with the avoidance of the various "refinements" advocated by certain enthusiasts. The "refinements" in question may doubtless intensify sexual pleasure for a time and even enhance sexual activity, but these advantages are paid for by an earlier extinction of normal sexual power. Still, though we regard as injurious many of the elements of the "art of love" as advocated by Van de Velde, we cannot but agree with this author that persistence in the regular practice of coitus, even by men well up in years, will help to postpone the onset of functional inactivity of the reproductive organs.

Impotentia Generandi

We have already explained that there may be incapacity for procreation, leading to sterility, in persons who have no difficulty in achieving complete intercourse—who are free from impotentia cœundi. Impotentia generandi may be partial or complete. For the moment we are considering males only, and are not concerned with the conditions which may make a woman comparatively infertile or wholly barren. Until recently, a rough and ready test was applied. When a marriage proved infertile the husband's semen (taken from a condom or from his wife's vagina very soon after the sexual act) was examined microscopically. If actively moving spermatozoa were present, it was assumed without more ado that the cause of the sterility of the pair must be sought in the female partner. Of late, however, the researches of Dr. Gerard L. Moench of New York City have put us on the track of a method whereby the degree of masculine fertility can be more accurately determined. It appears that absolute sterility in men is comparatively rare, but that the presence of motile spermatozoa in the semen is by no means a proof that the person concerned is competent for procreation. The chief cause of complete sterility in males is bilateral occlusion of the vasa deferentia in consequence of gonorrhœal epididymitis; but sterility can likewise result from chronic poisoning of various kinds and from nutritive disorders; it is also observed from time to time in men who in other respects seem perfectly normal.

Moench has made an extensive study of the shape and size of the head of the spermatozoon, and has discovered that in this way it is possible to detect the existence of diminished fertility in men whose semen contains actively moving spermatozoa. We will not here discuss the technique of the method, and will content ourselves with saying that it is likely to furnish results of practical value. Mönch has found reasons for believing that coitus interruptus, when persisted in, may prove extremely injurious to masculine fertility. It would also appear that when the fertility of the male is reduced, improvement may result in many cases from giving the generative organs a complete rest, in conjunction with measures for the improvement of the general health, vigorous bodily exercise, etc.

CHAPTER XVI

Sterility in Women

Not infrequently when a married couple remain without issue, skilled examination fails to discover in either of the partners anything to account for the barrenness. Especially perplexing are cases in which the childless husband and wife separate, to enter into fresh unions with partners who have likewise previously been barren, and find that in these new unions children are procreated. To account for such instances, people used to talk of an incompatibility between ovum and spermatozoon in the original union, or of something unsatisfactory in the reaction between the semen and the vaginal or cervical secretion, in the sterile marriages, or of mental causes of barrenness (a lack of adequate reciprocal desire). Such explanations are purely theoretical, lying beyond the range of scientific proof. Moench's investigations have thrown some light upon the possible causation. The sterility may have been due to a transient reduction in the fertilising power of the semen. As already said, full potentia generandi may be restored to the male by a considerable period of sexual abstinence, by improvement in the general health, by bodily exercise and careful attention to diet. That may account for the perplexing cases, or at any rate for some of them; but it must be admitted that the matter has not yet been fully cleared up.

Far more often, however, when a married woman remains childless, and when her sterility is not dependent upon the use of preventives, medical examination will disclose in her a sufficient cause for barrenness. In a good many cases sterile women whose reproductive organs are ostensibly normal and healthy will be found to exhibit an unmistakably " masculine " type of body. In such persons the lack of typical feminine characteristics is the expression of some abnormality in the ovarian or pituitary incretion, an abnormality which can be confidently assumed to exist although our present means of investigation are not sufficiently subtilised to enable us to detect any changes in the respective glands. At present, moreover, we know of no way in which sterility thus arising can be relieved. A more frequent cause of barrenness in women, however, is " infantilism ", a condition in which the woman's reproductive organs have failed to become fully adult, and thus to acquire the anatomical structure and the physiological functions fitting them for conception and gestation. In a good many cases of the kind the long-continued use of ovarian and pituitary extracts will lead to a proper development of the reproductive organs, and the previously barren women will become fertile. An ovarian graft (human), if it can be obtained and successfully implanted, is still more likely to be effective.

Very often the examination of a barren woman will show her to be suffering from chronic inflammation of the ovaries, the Fallopian tubes, or the uterus, usually as a sequel of gonorrhœal infection. Occasionally, in such cases, treatment will effect a cure. Other infections than gonorrhœa can unfit the uterus, the tubes, or the ovaries for the function of procreation. We frequently see cases in which a woman bears one child and thereafter remains sterile, as the outcome of an infective process which has spread upward from the vagina during childbirth. There are ways of discovering whether the Fallopian tubes are pervious, but they are not entirely free from risk, and their use should be left to gynæcological specialists.

Among additional causes of sterility in women may be mentioned tumours, displacements, and flexures of the uterus.

We have been able to give no more than a brief sketch of the multifarious causes of barrenness in women. Each case must be considered on its merits, and only a specialist can decide what is amiss. In concluding this chapter, we think it expedient to say that frigidity in women has little or nothing to do with sterility, as is proved by the fact that a woman who has been raped or to whom the act of sexual intercourse is disagreeable may readily become pregnant. Besides, frigidity is usually relative, for an absolute repugnance to sexual intercourse is rare. A woman may be frigid in intercourse with one man and may display a vigorous libido in intercourse with another. Marked, persistent, and general incapacity for sexual enjoyment is exceptional in women; and when it exists it is usually associated with the before-mentioned infantilism of the reproductive organs—which, as already said, can often be relieved by skilled treatment.

CHAPTER XVII

Abnormalities of the Sexual Life

General Considerations

It is customary to speak of those manifestations of the sexual impulse which differ from the ones manifested in normal relations between man and woman as perversions or aberrations. The most important of these must now be briefly described. We have to premise, however, that many noted authorities refuse, nowadays, to regard such unusual manifestations of the sexual impulse as morbid. Magnus Hirschfeld is the leader of a school of investigators who contend that the sexual impulse which draws man to woman and woman to man as the positive electron is attracted by the negative electron and, conversely, is not to be regarded as exclusively normal, nor are all divergent manifestations of the impulse to be stigmatised as pathological. These writers contend that the "typical" specimens of man and woman are but the extreme instances of a graded series. There are, it is held, numerous "intermediate stages" between the virile man and the feminine woman who are respectively a hundred per cent male and a hundred per cent female, and who can only find sexual gratification in union with the opposite type. Sexual relations, says Hirschfeld, are exceedingly multifarious, forming a series at one extremity of which is the "typical" man and at the other end the "typical" woman. In between come the manifestations (presently to be described) of sadism, masochism, transvestitism, exhibitionism, homosexuality, hermaphrodism, etc. These are regarded by Hirschfeld as intersexual types between that of the fully virile man and the fully feminine woman. Just as no two individuals are perfectly alike in aspect or in character, so, contends Hirschfeld, does the infinite variety of nature disclose itself in the manifold intermediate stages of sexual inclination and activity.

This is not the place for taking sides for or against the contention of Hirschfeld and his school, or for criticising their views from the outlook of those who continue to insist that what Hirschfeld terms " intersexuality " is the effect of an essentially morbid, and often curable, disorder of sexual sensibility. We shall content ourselves with adopting the classification of such phenomena to be found in Auguste Forel's excellent book *The Sexual Problem*—without prejudice as to whether what Hirschfeld calls " intersexual stages " are or are not to be regarded as morbid and abnormal. In concluding these introductory remarks, however, we must mention that whenever the sexual impulse is predominantly directed towards a person of the opposite sex it is termed " heterosexual " ; and whenever it is predominantly directed towards a person of the same sex it is termed " homosexual "

Perversions of the Heterosexual Impulse

Sadism and Masochism.—These two conditions are interrelated, and are jointly classed by Schrenk-Notzing under the comprehensive name of algolagnia, this meaning that sexual desire is attended by a longing to inflict or suffer pain—the sadist wishing to inflict pain, and the masochist to suffer it. (The pain may be either bodily or mental or both.) The sadist's sexual desire and sexual enjoyment are intensified by the suffering of the partner; the masochist's, by his own suffering. Both these terms are derived from the names of the persons who were the first to describe the aberrations in question, and who were themselves respectively affected by them. The Marquis de Sade (1740–1814) dilates upon a lascivious longing to humiliate, misuse, and in extreme cases even to kill the object of sexual love. Sacher-Masoch (1835–95), on the other hand, was affected by and described a sexual impulse accompanied by the longing to be humiliated and hurt by the beloved object. In a word, sadism is active algolagnia, and masochism is passive algolagnia. Forel points out, with good reason, that moderate degrees of algolagnia are not infrequently noticeable in connection with the normal sexual impulse. In like manner Brunner writes of sadism and masochism: "There is a trace of them in every love act, though it may be hidden away in the darker corners. As an accompaniment of a normal love relationship there occasionally ensues a moderate amount of beating and biting—which may be more than moderate in some of the lower animals. The tomcat sometimes bites the neck of his sexual partner; the male agouti treats the female in the same way; and among barndoor fowls the cock, when treading his hens, pecks them vehemently on the back of the head. There are such algolagniac components in the normal sexual intercourse of human beings, and what we call masochism is but a caricatured and exaggerated expression of normal passive algolagnia, the masochist feeling impelled towards extreme self-abasement and towards some symbolical (or even actual) suspension of the impulse towards self-preservation. The sadist, on the other hand, wishes to hurt, to bite, to scratch, to draw blood from his sexual partner; and in extreme cases this goes on to lust-murder and to anthropophagy, parts of the body being eaten. Even anthropophagy is but a morbid intensification of a loving impulse which normally finds expression in the exclamation: 'I love you so much that I should like to eat you!'"

From Brunner's abstract description of the nature of masochism and sadism, let us pass to consider the concrete manifestations of both. The justification for classing sadism and masochism together as algolagnia lies in this, that both may be simultaneously present in the same individual or may pass from one into the other. Still, marked and exclusive sadism or masochism is commoner than the mixed form of these perversions. A sadist is one who finds sexual gratification in the infliction of mental or bodily suffering upon the object of "affection", in humiliating and reviling, in whipping, in cutting or stabbing, in torturing with instruments which may be specially constructed for the purpose, and even in actual slaying. In such sadistic manifestations all grades may be noticed, ranging from the gentle love-bites previously described to the most abominable outrages. Conversely, a masochist finds sexual pleasure in suffering the very things which, when actively inflicted, give delight to the sadist. We have hitherto avoided the use of personal pronouns in speaking of these aberrations, for the reason that, although they may occur in both sexes, it would seem that a sadistic trend is perhaps more frequently manifested by women and a masochistic by men, while in homosexuals whether male or female either masochism or sadism may be present. We must not confuse with masochism as a perversion the inclination of women to play a passive part in normal sexual activity; and even though, in certain strata of society and especially in countries where civilization is at a low level, wives are often beaten by their husbands and perhaps expect to be maltreated in this way, we must not speak of such a manifestation as masochistic. There can be no question that masochism as a well-developed and indubitably morbid perversion of the sexual impulse—as a special type of sexual enjoyment—is rarer in women than in men. A special variety of masochism is what is known as flagellantism, by which we mean, not a sadistic desire to flog the sexual partner, but what may be termed "automasochism". The flagellant is usually one in whom a masochistic trend is associated with the morbid religious notion that self-chastisement will be pleasing to God and will help the person who thus tortures himself (or herself) to enter the kingdom of heaven. The sexual components of the flagellant impulse provide the key to the understanding of the morbid activities of many martyrs, fakirs, and other religious fanatics.

Fetishism.—In a fetishist (using that term in the sexual sense) the love-impulse, instead of being directed, as normally towards the whole organism and the integral personality, is diverted towards a portion of that personality, or, maybe, towards some lifeless physical object related to the chosen personality. One of the commonest forms of this fetishism is that in which a man is fascinated by a particular article of feminine wearing apparel. This is but an exaggeration and distortion of the normal. It is characteristic of the normal libido of the male that sexual desire is aroused in him by special parts of a woman's body, by articles of her clothing, by the aroma of her body, and even when no woman is actually present by the idea of the female reproductive organs. But to the fetishist the part has become greater than the whole. A shoe, a pocket-handkerchief, a glove, a tress of hair, a woman's hand or foot or breast, is no longer a subordinate part or symbol of a beloved woman, but seems an end in itself. The sight of the fetish, contact with it, the mere thought of it, will suffice to arouse sexual excitement. We have not space here to enumerate the multifarious forms of fetishism. It must suffice to mention the "plait cutters", persons who cut plaits of hair from the heads of young girls, who are happy in the subsequent possession of these plaits, and who obtain sexual gratification simply by looking at and touching them; and those very peculiar fetishists in whom sexual excitement can only be aroused by a woman who has a squint, or by one with a club-foot, or some other anomaly. Fetishism is far commoner in men than in women, and is found among homosexual as well as among heterosexual males.

Exhibitionism.—The typical male exhibitionist is one who has an impulse to expose himself in the presence of women. Such persons can only obtain gratification when observed by women. They never make any direct sexual assault; rather they tend to keep their distance, and readily take to flight. In women, well-marked exhibitionism is seen only in those suffering from grave mental disorder; and in men the exhibitionist trend is always the expression of a psychopathic taint, although obvious insanity is not necessarily present. Sooner or later an exhibitionist is likely to fall into the hands of the police, but punishment or the dread of it will not prevent his giving rein to his morbid impulse. Psychotherapy is worth a trial in such cases, but is often ineffective.

Homosexuality

Homosexuality is a comprehensive term to denote the direction of the sexual impulse towards persons of the same sex. In most cases it is associated with a disinclination for, and even a horror of, heterosexual activity. Heterosexual persons, the great majority, respond by regarding homosexuals as morbid or depraved; but homosexuals are inclined to regard themselves as a physiological variety, and even to speak of themselves as a "third sex". The view that homosexuals represent an intermediate sexual class, a transition between male and female, has of late years been put forward by the famous sexologist Magnus Hirschfeld. Moll considers them to be sick persons who can, often enough, be cured by psychotherapeutic methods.

Criminal statutes have had little or no effect in reducing the frequency of homosexual practices among those instinctively inclined to them. Unfortunately, the blackmailer has been the chief beneficiary of these statutes. By threatening exposure, and by playing upon his victim's dread of criminal prosecution, the blackmailer frequently reaps a golden harvest as he harries his prey to ruin, and even to suicide.

Worst, of course, among homosexual offenders are adults engaging in homosexual practices with the young and immature. Homosexuals themselves are prone to glorify their love for youths, and to remind us of the important part pædophilia played in the amatory life of ancient Greece. Moll points out, in a large proportion of homosexual adults the impulse is specially directed towards youths of an age ranging between fourteen and twenty. Herein lies danger. The present writers remain unconvinced by Hirschfeld's arguments that in the great majority of homosexuals their impulse is inborn, even though it be true that many of them exhibit a markedly feminine type associated with anomolies of the sexual secretions and of the reproductive organs.

It is unquestionable that in a fair proportion of homosexuals examination of the external reproductive organs during life or a post-mortem examination will disclose a varying degree of hermaphrodism. This anomaly, must, therefore, be considered.

Hermaphrodism

Hermaphrodism denotes the simultaneous occurrence of male and female reproductive organs, being the rule in most plants and in many of the lower animals. In human beings, however, individuals with perfectly developed male and female reproductive glands are extremely rare. Much commoner than such true hermaphrodism is pseudo-hermaphrodism, in which an individual has normal testicles or ovaries, but the other reproductive organs, external and internal, approximate more or less to the type proper to the opposite sex. In a fair proportion of male pseudo-hermaphrodites, notwithstanding the existence of testicles, the secondary sexual characters may be distinctively feminine. Such persons may have the wide hips of women, strongly developed breasts, feminine voices, and, above all, the emotional inclinations peculiar to women. Their counterparts are female pseudo-hermaphrodites. Such persons' external reproductive organs tend towards the masculine type, and their whole habit of body and secondary sexual characters may be decisively masculine. There are numerous transitions between these well-developed forms of pseudo-hermaphrodism. For instance, an individual whose organs are predominantly and unmistakably male or female in type, may exhibit one or two of the secondary sexual characters proper to the other sex. We come across men who have a woman's breasts; women whose larynx and voice are those of a man. Fairly common are women with a man-like growth of beard, or the hairy covering of the body in other respects similar to that of the male. With or without such obvious physical anomalies, the character may be "transitional". Fairly often we see persons whose external and internal reproductive organs and secondary sexual characters are those of a man or of a women, as the case may be, but who are unmistakably "inverted" in respect of tastes, modes of thought, and love inclinations. We may suppose that in such "intermediates", or in many of them, in some way not as yet fully understood, there have arisen anatomical changes in the reproductive mechanism owing to which the endocrine secretions, the hormones poured into the blood by the reproductive glands, have induced biochemical changes, and that consequently the persons concerned are instinctively and naturally impelled towards homosexual love. This being so, it would be absurd to expect, in all cases of homosexuality, that psychotherapy can restore a "normal", that is to say a heterosexual, mode of feeling.

In these matters the authors take a middle course. They find it impossible to accept the Freudian view that in the great majority of instances homosexuality is the outcome of a sexual trauma during early youth and can be cured by psychoanalysis. But they are equally reluctant to accept Magnus Hirschfeld's contention that no one can be seduced into homosexual ways of loving and into homosexual activities unless he or she is constitutionally predisposed towards homosexuality. It is generally admitted that during puberty and very early manhood or womanhood a considerable degree of ambivalence or bipolarity prevails in respect of the sexual impulse. Very numerous girls and a considerable proportion of youths pass through a phase of more or less "bisexuality", and during this period homosexual seduction which would at other times be inoperative may give the character a twist. No doubt we not infrequently encounter persons who during the period of bisexual vacillation are constitutionally inclined towards normal heterosexual activity, and yet may be misled into homosexual practices; at length, however, the heterosexual inclination may break through, to the subsequent exclusion of homosexuality. On the other hand, there are instances in which persons who by constitution are predisposed towards homosexuality, may fail to discover this inclination during the critical years of youth. A homosexual man may marry, live in seeming content with his wife, and have a number of children. Then, in the years of his maturity, he may become aware that he is a homosexual, and may suffer intensely from the conflict between his homosexual desires and the quasi-platonic affection which still persists for his wife and the mother of his children. If such a man enters into a homosexual liaison and then becomes the victim of a blackmailer, so that his social and economic position is endangered, his life becomes a hell.

We cannot refrain from insisting that in many cases homosexual inclinations are the outcome of a psychopathic constitution, and that for this and other reasons it is eminently undesirable that homosexuals should be given unrestricted opportunities for their propaganda among persons in the bisexual phase of youth.

It has been asserted by some that homosexual practices cannot possibly be the outcome of a psychopathic constitution seeing that some of the most distinguished men known to history were homosexuals. There is a flaw in the argument. It may be true that, to name only two famous instances, Leonardo da Vinci and Michelangelo, were homosexuals. But it is also likely enough that these great artists were bisexually inclined, for it must be remembered that the men of the Renaissance were inclined to make a cult of the feelings and practices, the thoughts and tastes, of classical antiquity, when the love of youths was a definite part of the sociological structure of the time. However this may be, the psychopathic inferiority of the average homosexual is not diminished by the fact that an occasional man of genius may have been inclined towards homosexual activities. Genius and insanity are interlinked in many ways, and geniuses are persons characterised by the supreme development of certain faculties whose less conspicuous manifestations in average persons of a similar constitutional type are apt to lead to lifelong confinement in a lunatic asylum. Kretschmer, the Marburg psychiatrist, has given a masterly description of the manic-depressive phases in the life and productivity of Goethe. In Emil Ludwig's *Goethe* we can also trace the periodicity in the poet's love life and mentality in a way which confirms the soundness of Kretschmer's view that genius (not Goethe's only) is, in all its manifestations, a particular phase or expression of the psychopathic taint. Manic-depressive insanity is not the less insanity because in some persons of manic-depressive constitution their peculiar temperament flames up into genius. It is precisely this flame of genius which was needed to account for the impressiveness of Goethe, who would otherwise have been nothing more than a privy councillor of Saxe-Weimar with his fluctuations to either side of the "normal", and with writings characterised by many incomprehensibilities and scurrilities. Even though many homosexuals have been talented, and a few have been persons of genius, the fact remains that psychopaths and hysterics predominate among persons with homosexual inclinations.

CHAPTER XVIII

A FEW WORDS ON THE HISTORY OF VENEREAL DISEASE

THE venereal diseases constitute those diseases which are mainly, though not exclusively, transmitted from person to person during the act of sexual intercourse. Until not so very long ago they were often lumped together as one "venereal disease". Their differentiation has been effected and a knowledge of their specific causes has been acquired only in comparatively recent years. At the present time we recognise four main venereal diseases: gonorrhœa, syphilis, the soft or non-infecting chancre (called "non-infecting" because it does not, like the "hard" chancre, which is the primary manifestation of syphilis, lead to a constitutional disease), and lymphogranulomatosis inguinalis. In the present volume we shall not give a detailed description of these various diseases, but must refer our readers to medical handbooks. All that we propose is, in the present chapter, to present a brief account of their history; and in the next chapter to discuss their individual prophylaxis (prevention).

Not in the Bible alone, but in the early literature of all peoples who have a literature—in the works of Indian, Japanese, Greek, and Roman writers—we find numerous references (mostly satirical) which show that the venereal diseases were known to the ancients. Several passages in the Old Testament indicate that gonorrhœa had come within the ken of some of its authors. The excavations at

Pompeii have shown that the use of bougies was known in classical Rome. Medieval writings manifest a fairly extensive acquaintance with gonorrhœa and many of its complications. We also find, in more ancient works, occasional references to ulcers of the reproductive organs. Still, at the close of the nineteenth century and in the early years of the twentieth, the general belief among experts was that syphilis is a comparatively modern scourge, not having existed either in antiquity or in the Middle Ages—as far, at any rate, as Europe is concerned. Of late, however, the view has come to prevail that syphilis is a much older disease than this, perhaps virulent to begin with, but then existing in a comparatively mild form, until, in the sixteenth century it became far more severe and manifested an epidemic prevalence—with the result that, like the influenza epidemic of the year 1918, it produced the impression of being a new disease.

We shall not attempt to decide whether the "antiquarian" school is right, or whether syphilis was brought back from the West Indies as one of the fruits of Columbus' first voyage. This much is certain, that the epidemic of syphilis began in 1493, the disease spreading from Spain, and manifesting itself in Italy with great virulence in the year 1495, after the taking of Naples by the mercenary soldiers of Charles VIII. Carried by the disbanded men to the various countries of Europe, it was also soon transported by the Portuguese to the Far East, to India, China, and Japan. The general symptoms of this widespread epidemic were exceedingly severe, taking the form of purulent and ulcerative processes in the skin, the bones, and the internal organs, and often proving fatal in the acute stage. Its virulence subsided towards the middle of the sixteenth century, and the disease came to assume the type with which we are nowadays familiar. Owing to the epidemic prevalence of this extremely severe form of syphilis, and owing to the conspicuousness of the primary ulcerative manifestations in the reproductive organs, gonorrhœa and chancroid, or soft chancre, passed into the background, and were, both by doctors and laymen, confounded with syphilis. For two centuries thereafter this " doctrine of identity " prevailed, syphilis, chancroid, and gonorrhœa being looked upon as different forms of one and the same disease. In the eighteenth century the famous British surgeon Hunter made an experiment which seemed to confirm the doctrine of identity. He inoculated himself with a secretion he believed to be gonorrhœal, and, as a result, he suffered from syphilitic infection. In the light of our present knowledge, we must suppose that the secretion used by Hunter in his experiments, though derived from the urethra, was not gonorrhœal, but was the discharge from a primary syphilitic sore hidden away within the urethra. It was not until the 'thirties of the nineteenth century that Philippe Ricord, a French investigator, succeeded in discrediting the hitherto dominant doctrine of the identity of " venereal disease ". He believed, and ere long the medical profession in general came to hold the view, that gonorrhœa, soft chancre, and hard chancre (the primary syphilitic sore), were caused by three distinct poisons. The question was not, however, set at rest until the science of bacteriology became well established. In 1879, Neisser discovered the gonococcus, the exciting cause of gonorrhœa ; in 1889, Ducrey identified the streptobacillus ulceris mollis, the organism which produces soft chancre; and finally, in the year 1905, Schaudinn, in joint work with E. Hoffmann, was able to show that the spirochæta pallida was the actual cause of syphilis. The organism of lymphogranulomatosis inguinalis, distinguished in the year 1923 as a fourth venereal disease, has not yet been identified.

CHAPTER XIX

Individual Prophylaxis

There is no absolutely trustworthy chemical substance which can safeguard against infection a man who has intercourse with a woman suffering from some form of venereal disease. As regards syphilitic infection, an ointment containing corrosive sublimate, prepared according to the formula of Neisser and Siebert, is probably the best available prophylactic (preventive of infection). It should, of course, be applied to the penis before intercourse. As regards the prevention of gonorrhœal infection, the installation into the urethra of a 2 per cent solution of silver nitrate will be likely to kill any gonococci that may have found their way into the canal, but this causes a good deal of smarting; so a 20 per cent solution of protargol in glycerine will be preferred. Various other preparations of silver salts and antiseptic ointments can be obtained from chemists as preventives of gonorrhœa, but, as already said, none of them are thoroughly dependable. They are most likely to be effective when used as soon as possible after intercourse.

Far more reliable than any chemical substance as a preventive of gonorrhœa is the wearing of a condom or sheath. If it does not tear, it will be an almost absolute safeguard—but it cannot, to the same extent, be trusted to ward off syphilitic infection. The spirochetes of syphilis can make their way through the most trifling fissures and abrasions in the skin, and can probably penetrate intact mucous membrane—that of the lips for instance. It therefore behoves a man who is careless in the choice of a sexual partner to remember the ease with which syphilitic infection can be brought about. All the same, the application of the Neisser-Siebert ointment to the penis before and after intercourse, or of some mercurial disinfecting ointment of a similar kind, gives a fairly efficient safeguard, the lubricating element of the ointment being helpful as well as the bactericidal (since a lubricated penis is less likely to suffer abrasion). It should be a general rule after a suspect coitus to pass water immediately and to wash the genital organs with soap and water and with a 1 per 1,000 sublimate solution. If there is no sublimate solution available, a thorough washing with soap and hot water may suffice to avert infection. Even when a condom has been used it will be well to wash this thoroughly with an antiseptic solution before removing it, or otherwise infection may still occur during the act of removal. A man who has had a suspect intercourse without having worn a condom will do well to consult a doctor as speedily as possible or to visit a disinfecting station—a public "Rettungswache" (in Germany). If more than twelve hours have elapsed, however, it will probably be too late to nip venereal infection in the bud.

Moreover, a man should never forget that, in all classes of society, there are plenty of unscrupulous women prepared to conceal the fact or even when questioned to deny that they are suffering from venereal disease. Furthermore, many women are in an infective condition without being aware of it. Sometimes a woman may erroneously suppose her illness to have been cured, but it is possible for the sufferer from venereal disease to be quite unaware of its existence. We must remember that during the period of incubation, which lasts for several weeks, a man who has been infected is a syphilitic without knowing it. It is far more easy for a woman to suffer in ignorance, as, for instance, when she has a primary syphilitic sore on the cervix uteri. Again, there are countless women who suffer for years from gonorrhœa without having their attention drawn to it by any well-marked symptoms. Far from uncommon are cases in which a married woman is infected immediately after marriage by her husband, a sufferer from an inconspicuous chronic gonorrhœa. This is the *Morgengabe*, the bridegroom's wedding-present to his bride! She may, quite innocently, remain unaware of the existence of this trouble until, having intercourse with another man, she infects him with the disease. Now, maybe, there will be a "light-up" of the trouble. Perhaps the vaginal mucous membrane had become tolerant of the gonococcus in a "mitigated" form. In her lover the organism may become virulent, and he may reinfect her with it in its virulent form. Then she may transmit this virulent gonorrhœa to her husband. In such cases the French speak of a "gonorrhée en trois".

Inasmuch as a man who frequently changes his sexual partner is always liable to venereal infection, the authors must be most emphatic in their warning that such a man must hasten to consult a physician directly he observes any local symptoms, whether in the way of urethral discharge or of what may seem to be a trifling pimple on the penis. It must never be forgotten that the earlier treatment of venereal disease is begun the better are the prospects of cure. Precious time is often wasted because the sufferer thinks that a little stickiness of the urinary meatus or a pimple on the penis is of no importance, and that the trouble will spontaneously disappear. It is disastrous, in such cases, for the patient to apply remedies of his own choosing or those recommended to him by lay friends. The only result will be to postpone an accurate diagnosis and to retard the beginning of effective treatment. For instance, although it is possible nowadays to diagnose syphilis with certainty at an early stage by the discovery of spirochetes in the primary sore, this early diagnosis will often be rendered impossible if, before coming to the doctor, the patient has been applying tincture of iodine, an antiseptic ointment, acetate of alumina, or lunar caustic—for these " remedies " will have driven the infective organisms from the surface into the deeper layers of the ulcer.

As regards a woman who has had sexual intercourse with an individual suspect of venereal disease, the possibilities of personal prophylaxis are less encouraging than in the case of the male. For the women, too, the best safeguard is that her male partner should wear a condom. Occasionally, maybe, an antiseptic vaginal douche immediately after intercourse may protect a woman from an attack of gonorrhœa which would otherwise ensue. In most cases, however, a man suffering from gonorrhœal infection will, in intercourse, infect the woman's urethra as well as her vagina, and in that case a vaginal douche will obviously be unavailing. In the case of both sexes, every act of intercourse must be regarded as suspect when the sexual partner is one inclined to promiscuity. Strict monogamy is, in fact, the best safeguard against the venereal diseases.

CHAPTER XX

Heredity

In human beings, as in all animals and plants that reproduce their kind sexually, the reproductive cells are the transmitters of hereditary qualities. It is through the instrumentality of these cells that certain qualities pass from parents to offspring. The reader has learned that in the cell nuclei of any species the number of chromosomes is constant, a doubling of the number of chromosomes in each successive generation being prevented by the " reduction division " which precedes the fusion of the nuclei of the ova and spermatozoa to form the fertilised ovum. According to our present lights, therefore, the chromosomes must be regarded as the actual bearers of heredity. Various names are used for the elements of the chromosomes in which hereditary qualities are incorporated. Thus we speak of heredity factors, idioplasm, genes, determinants, etc. For every hereditarily transmissible quality, the fertilised ovum must contain two determinants, one derived from each of the parents. According, however, to the nature and working of the determinants from the respective parents, an inherited character may be obvious or latent. When it is obvious, the character is said to be " dominant ", and when it is latent the character is said to be " recessive ". It is to Gregor Mendel (1822–84), Augustinian monk and subsequently prelate at Brünn, that we owe our first knowledge of the intimate laws of heredity.[1] Mendel's

[1] Cf. Iltis, *Life of Mendel*, London, 1932.

investigations date from the year 1864, but were little noticed at the time, and had lapsed into oblivion until, at the turn of the century, attention was drawn to them by the results obtained by other workers in the same field. Pursuing independent lines of inquiry, Tschermak, Correns, and de Vries happened upon the law discovered a generation before by Mendel as regards inheritance in the vegetable kingdom. Briefly formulated, what is now known as Mendel's Law runs as follows: If two varieties of animal or plant differing each from the other in respect of one character be crossed, the offspring of the first generation will almost all of them show the character as exhibited by one of the two parents, this being the dominant character, whereas the recessive character will seem to have disappeared. In the next generation, however, we find that one-fourth of the offspring exhibit the recessive character whereas three-fourths of them exhibit the dominant character. These generations are called respectively F^1 (the first filial generation) and F^2 (the second filial generation). If we continue our experiments we find that in the next generation, F^3 (the third filial generation), the hybrids can be grouped as follows: One-fourth of them manifest the dominant character exclusively, breeding true in this respect in successive generations; one-fourth of them in like manner exhibit the recessive character exclusively, and breed true in this respect; but the remaining two-fourths are like the hybrids of the F^2 generation, being themselves hybrids which segregate once more in accordance with the ratios 1 : 2 : 1.

A specific example will make this clearer. In the plant known as marvel of Peru, four o'clock or Mirabilis jalapa, there are two well-marked varieties, one bearing white flowers and the other red flowers. If we cross a white-flowering and red-flowering four o'clock, the hybrids of the F^1 generation all have pink flowers. Inbreeding from the pink-flowering plants of this F^1 generation, we get an F^2 generation in which two-fourths of the specimens have pink flowers, one-fourth white flowers, and one-fourth red flowers. If we now inbreed from the white-flowering plant of the F^2 generation and separately from the red-flowering plant of the F^2 generation, we shall find that these breed true, red-flowering and white-flowering respectively, for an indefinite number of generations; but if we inbreed from the pink-flowering plant of the F^2 generation, which constituted two-fourths of the specimens, we find that their offspring segregate once more in the same proportion as did the hybrids of the previous generation into white-flowering, pink-flowering, and red-flowering plants. Thus, taking into consideration all the plants of the F^2 generation, we are able, after studying their behaviour in the next, F^3, generation, to divide them into three groups. One-fourth of them manifest the dominant character exclusively, breeding true in this respect in successive generations; one-fourth of them, in like manner, exhibit the recessive character exclusively, and breed true in this respect; but the remaining two-fourths are like the hybrids of the F^1 generation, being themselves hybrids which segregate once more in accordance with the ratios 1 : 2 : 1. From generation to generation, therefore, the number of pink-flowering plants will decrease, while the number of white-flowering and red-flowering plants will increase. The plants which breed true, those which in our example produce always white flowers or red flowers, have completely lost one of the determinants of the hybrid characters, the white-flowering plant having lost the determinant that produces red flowers, and the red-flowering plant having lost the determinant that produces white flowers. Such plants are spoken of as "homozygotic", whereas the hybrids containing both the red-flower and the white-flower determinant (therefore, in the case of the four o'clock, producing pink flowers) are said to be "heterozygotic". We have seen, however, that half of the offspring of the heterozygotic hybrids have once more become homozygotic.

It follows from these experiments that, during the fusion of the respective nuclei of the ovum and the spermatozoon, or, in the case of plants, of ovum and pollen, the determinants, genes, or heredity factors derived from the respective parents must remain distinct. In the foregoing example, the red-flower determinant and the white-flower determinant do not fuse, either in the nucleus of the fertilised ovule, or in the cells which are produced by its division and redivision. In the F^1 generation of four o'clock, all the plants contain both determinants, and the flowers are therefore pink instead of being either red or white; but in the subsequent filial generations the red-flower determinant and the white-flower determinant, being only loosely connected, undergo segregation in half of the offspring. We have here taken a very simple case, and concerning one character only. The general course of heredity is greatly complicated by the fact that in the germ-plasm the determinants of all kinds of qualities are very variously mingled, and that some of them being dominant and others being recessive they influence the characters of the offspring in the most diversified way. It would take us too far beyond the scope of the present work to follow this topic further. We cannot here go into further details concerning the way in which these researches have been extended, or concerning the far-reaching hypotheses that are now being formulated about heredity. We will, however, make a brief reference to the remarkable fact of mutation, discovered by de Vries. This investigator showed that hereditary characters may suddenly disappear or newly appear in living beings.

As regards human heredity, the following important conclusions can be drawn from Mendel's Law. In the case of a fair number of diseases and predispositions to disease the nature of their heredity has now been ascertained, and it is possible to decide whether particular hereditary characters are, in the mendelian sense, dominant or recessive. For instance, almost all inheritable malformations and also diseases of the skin and disorders of metabolism (tissue change) in so far as inheritable, are dominant characters; whereas it would seem that the heredity factors inducing mental disorders are recessive. A recessive taint will not become manifest unless this particular taint exists in both parents. For example, if a person not ostensibly diseased but affected by inheritance with a transmissible hereditary taint (a recessive predisposition to mental disorder) marries a person of healthy stock, the recessive taint will not become manifest in their offspring, but may continue to be transmitted from generation to generation until at length one of the tainted stock marries a person whose stock bears the same recessive taint. Thereupon, although both of the parents have been free from mental disorder, such a disorder will manifest itself in their offspring.[1] It is therefore incumbent upon all persons whose forefathers have suffered from mental disorder to inquire, when contemplating marriage, whether there have been any manifestations of mental disorder in the ancestry of the proposed partner. Such questions as this, and those that concern hereditary diseases in general, form a proper subject of inquiry for marriage-advice bureaus (Eheberatungsstellen). Although many of the elements of the science of heredity still remain hypothetical, enough is already known to make it desirable that before marriage a careful inquiry should be made into the family history of the proposed partner. Where there is considerable probability that a contemplated union would result in the production of offspring with defective mental or bodily health, common sense and elementary morality forbid the proposed marriage. Closely connected with these ideas are the endeavours to apply our knowledge of heredity in the way of a deliberate selection of sexual partners in the hope of improving the race. Here we enter the field of eugenics, which will be considered in the next chapter.

[1] Cf. Baur, Fischer, and Lenz, *Human Heredity*, London, 1931.

CHAPTER XXI

EUGENICS AND RACIAL HYGIENE

THE apostles of eugenics and racial hygiene wish to subordinate reproduction to the deliberate and purposive control of the human will. The favouring of procreation by persons regarded as especially fine specimens of the race is termed "positive eugenics", and the hindering of procreation by inferior specimens is termed "negative eugenics". In the present state of our knowledge and in the extant social system, there are more extensive possibilities in the domain of negative than in that of positive eugenics. It is certainly possible—by castration, or by ligature of the vasa deferentia or the Fallopian tubes—to prevent the insane, epileptics, habitual criminals, etc., from reproducing their kind. An "Act to Prevent the Procreation of Confirmed Criminals, Idiots, Imbeciles, and Rapists" was approved by the legislature in Indiana on March 9, 1907, and since then similar acts have been placed on the statute book and enforced by a number of the States of the American Union. Objections to the compulsory sterilisation of epileptics, the insane, drunkards, etc., have been raised by persons who contend that such individuals classed as "defective" have often been the parents of geniuses. All the same, there is something to be said for the idea that the race will be improved by the exclusion of certain undesirable elements from reproduction.

Positive eugenics is the counterpart of negative eugenics,

its aim being that men and women should, by a wise choice of sexual partners, endeavour to increase the number of persons who are the bearers of what are regarded as exceptionally good hereditary trends. A good many of the advocates of positive eugenics are opposed to birth-control, to a deliberate restriction of the number of offspring. At the Congress for Sexual Reform at Copenhagen in the year 1928 Leunbach declared that eugenists could not but be horrified at the way in which the best types of our race were restricting their families or having no children at all while inferior types were propagating their kind without restraint. But, as we have already pointed out, under existing economic conditions (in Germany and elsewhere) it is futile to preach a doctrine of fecundity to those who have ears to hear. The better types, precisely because they are intelligent and have a keen sense of responsibility, will shrink from procreating many children in a world where poverty is rife. Not until, through a deliberate restriction of births, standing-room has been gained in the world, not until after this period of transition, will philoprogenitiveness—a fairly widespread instinct—be given free rein once more. Meanwhile, there is certainly work for the eugenists, although their gloomy vaticinations concerning the widespread multiplication of the unfit and their fears that the practice of birth control by the better types and races will lead to the disappearance of these, cannot but remind us a little of the way in which doctors recommend poverty-stricken consumptives to visit some Swiss health resort. In other words, eugenics as a practical policy can only be taken seriously when social conditions are so far improved that intelligent human beings will be able to count upon satisfactory material conditions and healthy surroundings, and a proper mental environment for the children they bring into the world.

One "negative eugenic" recommendation, however, being immediately realisable, though as yet to a large extent ignored, deserves widespread attention, namely the avoidance of the marriage of near kin. Experience teaches that breeding in and in, the marriage of persons who have numerous ancestors in common, has, as contrasted with the marriage of persons not connected by ties of blood, a tendency to produce offspring suffering from many morbid taints. For instance, night-blindness due to inflammation of the retina (retinitis pigmentosa) is especially common in the children of blood relations. Colour-blindness, again, and various malformations, are seen chiefly among the children of those who are closely related. The prevalence of glaucoma and retinitis pigmentosa in Jews seems to be in large measure dependent upon the close inbreeding of the Jewish population which has gone on for many centuries. The same thing accounts for the exceptional prevalence of mental disorder among Jews. The frequency of these and other hereditary diseases in the children of first cousins shows that there is plenty of scope for eugenic propaganda in this field.

When one of the partners of a proposed marriage is suffering from tuberculosis, and still more when both are affected with the disease, the desirability of avoiding such a union must be very seriously considered. We do not mean to imply that no tubercular patient should ever marry. Often enough the disease is so mild and so readily curable that a general prohibition of the marriage of the tubercular would appear to be unwarrantable. The disease is not itself inheritable[1]; but the predisposition to acquire it can certainly be transmitted, and is especially liable to be transmitted when both the partners suffer from hereditary taint. The children of such persons will be likely to have a peculiarly susceptible constitution, to exhibit what is technically known as a phthinoid (long and narrow) chest, and will be very readily infected with tuberculosis. Matters are made worse, of course, when the disease is active in either parent or in both, inasmuch as in such cases exposure to infection is persistent. Skilled advice should, therefore, always be sought before marriage by those known to suffer from a hereditary predisposition to tuberculosis, and still more by those in whom the disease is actively present. It must not be forgotten that in a woman suffering from tuberculosis, perhaps in a mild form, there is a great likelihood that the disease may become far more active during the stresses of pregnancy, childbirth, and lactation, with results exceedingly dangerous both to mother and to child.

Where both the parties to a proposed marriage are hereditarily inclined to extreme neurasthenia or to hysteria, eugenist considerations should lead us to advise against the union. Above all is this the case when there has been pronounced mental disorder in the family history of both parties. It can hardly be expected that the law will ever intervene in such matters. The best that can be hoped for is that eugenist propaganda will direct popular attention to the subject and will arouse a general willingness to abstain

[1] This statement would be challenged by some modern authorities—Lumière, for instance.—TRANSLATORS' NOTE.

from childbearing on the part of persons suffering from dangerous hereditary taints. The law could, however, usefully intervene by insisting upon the exchange of health certificates as a preliminary to marriage. This would at least have an educational influence. The arousing of a due sense of responsibility would doubtless be a slow process. It has taken thousands of years for the extant moral repugnance to incest to become firmly established. In the Homeric poems and in the sagas of all nations we find ample evidence that sexual unions between brothers and sisters were formerly regarded as perfectly reasonable and legitimate. It follows, therefore, that in the course of ages there may occur a change in popular sentiment whereby certain manifestations of the sexual impulse can be brought under control. Upon this change in popular sentiment we have to depend. The State cannot coerce nature; it can only help to disseminate knowledge, can only exert an educational influence. Working in this direction, the State must rely upon the observations and experiments of scientists, must avoid preconceived opinions, and must learn to interpret natural laws without prejudice.

Forel introduced the term blastophthoria (damage to the germ) to denote the effect of certain influences which he believed capable of directly injuring the germ-plasm and its chromosomes. According to Forel there are environmental influences which can injure the human reproductive cells before conjugation occurs, such "blastophthoria" producing the semblance of hereditary disease, whereas genuine hereditary disease is the outcome of determinants, some dominant and others recessive, existing in the ancestral germ-plasm and not due to environmental influences. Forel believed, however, that heritable disorders could be originated by blastophthoria, the germ cells damaged by environmental influences before conjugation being modified in a way that would subsequently be hereditarily transmissible. Special stress was laid by Forel upon this notion of blastophthoria in connection with the effects of the abuse of alcohol. He held that the spermatozoa and the ova of alcoholics were damaged by the poison circulating in their blood, and that the children of alcoholics were, therefore, likely to be idiots, epileptics, dwarfs, and so on. But the damage, he insisted, is not confined to the first filial generation; the blastophthoric idiots, epileptics, dwarfs, etc., in whom the trouble has been produced by alcoholism in the father or the mother or both, will be likely, even though they themselves are lifelong abstainers, to have weak-minded or epileptic offspring. The germ-plasm has been permanently damaged and a hereditary taint has been established. Since Forel formulated this theory a good many years ago, a considerable amount of evidence has accumulated in support of the contention that alcohol exerts a blastophthoric influence. There are good reasons, therefore, for advising very strongly against even a moderate indulgence in alcohol at the time of or shortly before procreation. The convention according to which, at a wedding feast, large quantities of alcohol are consumed, not only by the guests, but by the bridegroom and the bride, must be emphatically condemned from the eugenic standpoint. The recent experiments of Erwin Baur, Goldschmidt, and others have shown that various poisons besides alcohol, and also Röntgen rays, etc., are capable of inducing marked changes in hereditary qualities and of engendering new ones. The general upshot of these considerations is to throw doubt upon the alleged inalterability of the germ-plasm, upon the supposed inviolability of hereditary qualities.

Furthermore, from the outlook of sexual ethics, alcohol plays, in general, a sinister rôle—that of seducer and procuress. Sexual misdemeanours of all kinds are closely connected with the abuse of alcohol; and even very small quantities of this intoxicant, especially in persons who are exceptionally sensitive to its influence, will blunt the keen edge of moral restraint. Alcohol being a narcotic as well as a stimulant, will lead the drinker to forget or to underestimate the dangers of venereal infection. As a stimulant it increases sexual desire, but as an anæsthetic it usually causes a marked diminution of sexual enjoyment. A large dose may cause temporary impotence. "It provokes the desire, but it takes away the performance"—as the porter says in *Macbeth*. Day after day, numberless young men in a condition of very slight alcoholic intoxication forget all their good resolutions and enter into sexual relations with women they would certainly never dream of approaching but for the way in which their fine sensibilities have been dulled by liquor. In like manner a woman who is no more than a little "hilarious" will, in this condition, heedlessly give herself to a man. Innumerable and tragical are the instances in which, thanks to alcohol the seducer and procuress, venereal infection or an unwanted pregnancy has resulted. It is probable, indeed, that a majority of attacks of venereal disease have originated thanks to the co-operation of alcohol, seldom consumed to great excess, but merely taken in a quantity sufficient to make the person concerned feel cheerful and enterprising.

Obviously, then, the effects of alcohol are disastrous, both in respect of its influence upon the offspring (hereditary or pseudo-hereditary disease) and in respect of causing a dangerous unrestraint in the matter of sexual relationships. It is, too, a matter of common knowledge that alcohol is the main buttress of prostitution and criminality. We cannot, however, for these reasons endorse the recommendation that the State should unreservedly prohibit the use of alcoholic beverages. At all times among all nations intoxicants of one sort or another have been customarily used. The " strong arm of the law " has never been strong enough to eradicate such indulgences ; and the experiences of " prohibition " in the United States of America have been of a kind to give cause for reflection to all who might otherwise have been inclined to extend its blessings to European nations. Education, a gradual change in popular sentiment whereby alcoholic indulgence will be discountenanced for young persons and for all those in whom liquor is prone to induce sexual libertinage, are far more likely to be effective than the " axe " of prohibition. Just as the unwearied efforts of medical practitioners have of late years made university students realise that gonorrhœa is by no means a trifling ailment and should not be looked upon as a sort of certificate of the attainment of manhood, so in respect of alcoholic indulgence we must look for betterment to progressive educational work in conjunction with enhanced interest in sport and bodily exercise.

CHAPTER XXII

Advice Concerning Marriage

The marriage-advice bureaus which [in Germany] have of late years been established thanks to the efforts of those who set a high value upon social hygiene, will only be useful in the long run if the average man and the average woman come to regard the staffs of these places (medical practitioners of both sexes) as persons free from doctrinaire prejudices and competent to harmonise their aspirations for social welfare with a due regard for the personal happiness of those who seek their advice. The advisers who, in any particular case, recommend that a marriage should be entered into and see no reason for regarding it as undesirable, must never forget that even the acme of professional skill in conjunction with far-reaching knowledge of the world and of human character will never enable us to forsee the multifarious complications that may arise during the many years of married life. The advisers must therefore be content to study the clinical history and the family history of the partners to the proposed marriage, with a special eye to the possibility of recessive taints, and must, when necessity arises, utter emphatic warnings as to the risk and perhaps the certainty that the offspring, if there be any, will suffer from hereditary disease. Some eugenists contend that when both parties to a proposed marriage suffer from an identical hereditary taint, the marriage should not be prevented. Here, they say, are persons with a recessive and therefore hidden pathogenic trend. If we advise against the union, and our advice be accepted, the persons concerned will, sooner or later, marry someone else, and the recessive trend will persist in their offspring. Is it not better that the persons concerned should marry, with a view to the " mendelising out " of the disease, as practised by the breeders of plants and animals? The offspring of such a union should, of course, be sterilised (by ligature of the vasa deferentia or the Fallopian tubes). In that way, declare these remarkable philanthropists, the morbid taint in question could slowly but surely be eradicated from the human stock, and the quality of the race could be steadily improved. We regard a detailed criticism of such fantasies as superfluous. We cannot influence the operations of nature in her " breeding retorts " by measures whose naivety indicate that the fancies of the medieval alchemists still persist among us, notwithstanding the advance of modern science.

As a matter of fact, we do not believe that the marriage advisers will be able to do very much to induce individuals to refrain from marriage because the offspring of the proposed union will be, presumably, diseased or otherwise undesirable. Still, in view of the contemporary spread of the birth-control movement, they will doubtless be able, in many such instances, to emphasise the need for contraception when contraception is eminently desirable in the public interest. In this way the marriage-advice bureaus will do invaluable work by reducing the frequency of inborn defects, weaknesses, and diseases. Another useful field of activity for these bureaus will be the detection of preconjugal venereal disease in persons whose trouble has not been thoroughly cured, and who require further medical treatment. Alcoholics, consumptives, psychopaths, and drug addicts can also be advised to seek skilled treatment.

It may be hoped, then, that the marriage-advice bureaus will ultimately develop into State or municipal institutions at which, as at Norman Haire's birth-control clinic in London, working-class women will be instructed in the proper use of the methods of birth-control. They will further, in due time, become the organising centres in which the inducing of abortion can be advised when absolutely necessary for social or eugenic reasons. (This, of course, when the law concerning abortion has been reformed.) The child in the mother's womb is not exclusively her personal property, like her teeth, her hair, or her thoughts. It is the outcome, not of the impulse to self-preservation, but of the impulse to species preservation, of the self-love of the species, and therefore does not belong to the vessel which the species has chosen, to the particular woman's body in which the offspring is developing. Consequently the State, as an embodiment of the super-individual egoism of the species, has (in our opinion) over-riding rights in the control of the child, which is the product of the self-love of the species. But the State has duties as well as rights. It is the duty of the State to ensure that there shall be equally satisfactory possibilities of upbringing for all the newborn embodiments of the communal will. Under extant social conditions, the State does not fully recognise this duty, and is not in a position to fulfil it. It can, however, at least strive to achieve a compromise between its desire for a sufficiency of suitable offspring whereby the persistence of the species can be maintained, on the one hand, and its incapacity to provide satisfactory conditions of upbringing for all the members of the community, on the other.

In practice, therefore, the State cannot leave it to the individual pregnant woman to have abortion procured when, how, and where she pleases. It must provide, as Soviet Russia already provides, institutions at which abortion can be induced by experts, not only when the continuance of the pregnancy would endanger the mother's health, but also when no adequate economic provision for the upbringing of the child is forthcoming, when the existence of hereditary taint makes it almost certain that the offspring will be diseased, when the pregnancy has been the outcome of rape, of the seduction of a girl under age, and so on. The procuring of abortion at the caprice of the individual mother, and by unskilled hands or in other places than the authorised institutions, should, in our opinion, remain a punishable offence.

We believe that the reform here advocated would lead to a marked decline in poverty and human suffering, and would be followed by the development of a generation of human beings among whom, owing to the healthiness of their hereditary constitutions, the spectre of the falling birthrate and the dread of the dying-out of the population would have been laid to rest. It seems likely enough that, in due course, the marriage-advice bureaus will become the centres at which the desirability of inducing abortion will be determined. It is in this direction, we opine, that their usefulness will develop (perhaps in days that are still far distant); whereas it seems to us that the likelihood remains small that many persons will be influenced by their advice as regards the choice of a partner. One who believes that lovers will listen to advice, knows nothing of the nature of love! It is otherwise as regards the counselling of persons who are no longer passionate lovers but ordinary married folk, so that, as Brunner puts it, they have ceased to be a couple whose egoism has been fused in the crucible of the passion for species preservation, and have become persons whose thoughts and feelings, severed once more, move in the ambit of primitive, individualist egoism. Unless a strong intellectual tie persists, with a community of interests, economic or social, or perhaps a joint affection for the children, it is likely enough that, when the initial fervour of love due to the impulse towards species preservation has cooled, many a husband and many a wife will be in need of kindly counsel. Here the marriage-advice bureaus will certainly be able to fulfil a useful function, provided that they are staffed by persons of the right sort. When those who have been lovers and are now "merely husband and wife" no longer have any intrinsic ties, it will have to be frankly admitted that extrinsic considerations cannot be regarded as sufficient for desiring the persistence of a marriage which has ceased to be a true marriage. The demand for easy and speedy divorce in such instances is a reasonable one, and general compliance with it is only a question of time.

CHAPTER XXIII

Monogamy

In the concluding chapter of this work we wish to express our views as to what kind of sexual impulse and what kind of sexual life are best both for the individual and for the community. In the previous chapters, the authors have, indeed, frequently found occasion to emphasize their outlooks regarding love as a natural phenomenon and regarding the union of the sexes as a sociological and cultural manifestation. Now the time has come for a comprehensive statement of their position with regard to the problems of marriage and sexual reform—problems concerning which the contemporary world is greatly exercised and which have of late years been widely discussed in speech and in writing.

Just as the character varies greatly from individual to individual, and just as temperament and constitutional predisposition are extremely diversified, so likewise is erotic differentiation widespread throughout our species, making it difficult, if not impossible, to say what is "sexually normal". While it is true that all human beings, as egoists, tend to think and act under stress of certain powerful impulses (amative, possessive, acquisitive, self-assertive, etc.), while it is true that the longing for self-preservation animates them all, this fundamental tone is so infinitely modified by the diversity of the overtones as between one person and another, that no rules concerning what is most desirable for the conduct of the sexual life in men and in women can be prescribed by any authority. The best that can be hoped for is to formulate certain ideal demands, arrived at by the application of our extant scientific knowledge in such a way as to present what seems most desirable for the majority of the members of human society—for the mutual welfare of individuals and of society at large. Like all such ideals, it is something we shall be able to strive towards without ever wholly attaining. But the recognition that there is an ideal and the unceasing attempt to attain it seem to us indispensable. What, then, is the ideal in this matter of sexual behaviour?

To the present writers it seems beyond dispute that a monogamic union must be the sexual ideal of the normal human being. They agree with Marañon that: "The only successful solution for the unrest of the instincts is furnished by the couple bound together in love. . . . A man, no doubt, may find happiness in polygamy, of which the world offers numberless examples. . . . But such happiness can only be secured at the cost of the suffering and the shame of countless women. This being so, the first and most obvious solution, based upon sexual and individual egoism, is one which proves unacceptable. A woman who cannot be content to live in sexual ties with one man only, must either become a barren ascetic or else a Messalina; and she cannot become a Messalina without the collaboration of unworthy men."

In view of such considerations, we differ strongly from those "sexual reformers" who would sweep away the difficulties that arise because men are on the whole more polygamously inclined than women whereas women are on the whole more monogamously inclined than men, by conceding to women a right to polyandric activities just as men have claimed for themselves and have exercised polygamous activities—with the result that promiscuity, more or less, would become established as the ideal of sexual behaviour for our time. We hold that (to say nothing of morality) such a solution is unnatural and must be condemned from the biological standpoint. The natural calling of a woman has been, is, and must remain reproduction and the care of the offspring. Even though we do not accept the evolutionary doctrine in accordance with which mankind stands " highest " in the animal kingdom and is the crown of creation, still it seems to us that for the human species sexual promiscuity or polyandric activities on the part of women would signify a kind of degeneration. The discrepancy between the comparatively polygamous instincts of the male and the comparatively monogamous instincts of the female of the human species can be bridged over in a much simpler way and in one which will be perfectly innocuous to our race. It is easy enough for men (at any rate for the preponderant majority of men), and by no means unwholesome, to curb their polygamous impulses out of love for their comparatively monogamous sexual partner. The " double standard of sexual morality ", in accordance with which men were free to follow any prompting of erotic impulse while women were forbidden to do the same thing, has always been repulsive to decent-minded persons. In view of the position now attained by women and of the granting of equal rights to their sex, the struggle against the tradition of the double standard of sexual morality would appear to be a natural and necessary endeavour to abolish the last vestiges of the thraldom of women, to sweep away the last reminiscences of times when a woman was no more than the chattel of an irresponsible owner. But, as an outcome of this justified struggle against the double standard, to assign to women the right hitherto claimed and exercised by men in sexual matters, seems to us (we speak as biologists and not as moralists) sure to bring disaster in its train. The proper solution is the abandonment of masculine libertinage.

In a word, there is no warrant for the generalisation that men must be permitted occasional lapses from the monogamic code and that women must tolerate such lapses; and there is still less warrant for establishing a general right to an occasional change of partners or to unconditional libertinage both for men and for women. No doubt in special cases, above all when the sexual partners are of artistic temperament and are very highly differentiated persons, a union in which the bond is sustained by a community or egoistic or intellectual interests may continue to run a fairly harmonious course while each partner tolerates occasional sexual vagaries on the part of the other. Speaking generally, however, if the recommendation of a good many modern writers be followed, and if the monotony of marriage be tempered by occasional "passades" (in plain terms, by polygamous activities indulged in by both the partners of a reputedly monogamic union)—the almost invariable result will be that, sooner or later, such a marriage will break up. For what is marriage? It is a community entered into by a male egoist and a female egoist upon the foundation of reciprocal sexual attraction. As Brunner writes: "It only becomes a genuine marriage through a profoundly intimate coalescence of their respective egoisms, thanks to which neither of the egoists thus united will any longer regard his or her egoism as peculiar to himself or herself, seeing that both will look upon it as a joint egoism." Brunner, however, goes on to say that the sexual constitution of the male human being is such that when a married man seeks sexual gratification with another woman than his wife, he does not break up the "marriage" but only the "love bond" between himself and his wife—and the contention that he breaks up the marriage is an error arising from a mistaken identification of marriage with sexual love. Brunner holds that marriage imposes the obligation of monogamy upon the woman alone, and that she, indeed, breaks up the marriage as well as severing the love tie when she enters into relations with another man than her husband, inasmuch as she is not only a wife false to a husband, but a mother false to her children.

Although, in general, we share Brunner's views regarding the nature of love and of marriage, upon this point we differ from him. We do, indeed, agree that polygamous aberrations on the part of a husband are less serious than polygamous aberrations on the part of a wife. It lies in the nature of things that a wife should more readily tolerate and forgive a husband's infidelity than a husband a wife's; and, besides, it seems to us that infidelity on the part of the wife is far more dangerous to the integrity of the family than infidelity on the part of the husband. It seems probable, too, that there are still plenty of women who are quite indifferent to a husband's occasional infidelities. Still, the logical outcome of a demand that women should enjoy equal freedom with men in sexual behaviour would be that for women no less than for men infidelity would signify no more than a severing of the love tie and would not break up the marriage. The general upshot would be disastrous to the community at large. Even though it be true that a man's personality is less profoundly influenced than a woman's by occasional extra-conjugal indulgence, it must not be overlooked that, for the very reason that a woman is more monogamously inclined than a man, she will be apt to find it an outrage that her husband should seek the embraces of another woman.

This desire for exclusive possession is based upon a sound instinct, and in part upon a desire to check the spread of the venereal diseases. Other considerations apart, it is in the majority of instances a grave danger to marriage and to happiness in marriage that husbands, in their eagerness for sexual variety, should ignore the danger of contracting a venereal disease and then transmitting it to their wives. We therefore consider that the only right course is to move steadily towards the attainment of a genuine monogamy, and that this can only be achieved through the voluntary renunciation of polygamous activities on the part of men. No doubt Marañon is right when he declares that the proportion of married couples able to achieve permanent and complete monogamy is still comparatively small. All the same, genuine monogamy remains the only sound ideal for the future of mankind. The more the endeavour towards sexual differentiation is refined and ennobled, the more it is "sublimated", the less will sex as such be the exclusive force of attraction. A man will seek, instead of the mere embodiment of sexual characters, "an individual, a woman, who will incorporate the counterpart of his own peculiarities, of his own highly specialised masculine instincts." (Marañon.)

Monogamy being in our view the ideal form of marriage both for men and for women, we must obviously condemn the various forms of modified marriage which have been recommended of late years. As regards unregulated promiscuity, enough has already been said in condemnation of this as incompatible with civilisation. Passing on to consider various schemes which, while to some extent allowing marriage to persist in its present form, make allowance in varying degrees for the polygamous instincts of men and for polyandric indulgence on the part of women, we may mention, first of all, schemes for "triangular" marriage. (Some "sexual reformers" advocate a "quadrangular" marriage, and more than a hundred years ago Schopenhauer penned an essay on "tetragamy"; while others advocate group marriage on a larger scale.) Our comment on such schemes is that an interweaving of the egoistic interests of two human beings becomes impossible when a third partner is introduced, and still more when several additional partners are introduced, into this bond that is to be the expression of a most intimate community of bodily and mental interests. The advocates of triangular marriage, of tetragamy, and of group marriage, will not, however, be able to deny that the care and education of the offspring and the ethics of family life are already imperilled to a grave degree in our extant social order. Nor do we think that the "companionate" marriage advocated by Lindsey as a form of trial marriage is likely to prove advantageous. We have no more than a second-hand knowledge of Lindsey's views, but we understand that in what he terms a companionate the marriage of a young man and a young woman would be rendered possible by the supplementing of the man's income through allowances from the parents or through the joint earnings of the young wife provided always that the bearing of children should be postponed until the family income became large enough to allow of their proper upbringing. What is this but early marriage in the form which is now practically universal—with the disadvantages of trial marriage superadded? The so-called "week-end marriage" in which the couple do not live together, but meet for sexual relations each week-end, may also be mentioned here. It is of course a contradiction of terms to speak of this as "marriage" at all. It is nothing more than a fugitive love union, a variety of the "intimacy" or "liason", which may in exceptional instances prove successful enough to lead to a real marriage.

The present writers are, on the other hand, in sympathy with the sexual reformers' demand for an increased facility of divorce. It is self-evident that the partners in a really unhappy marriage must be enabled to separate more easily than has hitherto been possible. Only those who misunderstand the essential nature of marriage, can fail to recognise that the fusion of the egoistic interests of the partners to form a new joint interest must be fundamentally voluntary, and that it is preposterous that two persons should be forced to live together in conjugal relations maintaining the semblance of joint interests for which a spiritual substratum no longer exists. In many cases, certainly, though not perhaps in all, the abandonment of bodily relations between the pair must be followed by a complete severance of the conjugal tie.

In conclusion we wish, at the cost of repetition, to make it perfectly clear that when we speak of " marriage " we are not thinking only of a union that has been sanctioned by religion or by the State. Free-spirited and steadfast persons can, at times, sustain a conjugal union by voluntary agreement. Obviously, however, for most persons their own interests and those of the community at large will best be safeguarded by the official recognition of the union, were it only for legal reasons and with an eye to the inheritance of property. Even in Soviet Russia, marriage is still a union registered by the State, is still an officially recognised institution. Indeed, marriage as an officially recognised institution must remain part of the most essential foundation of any kind of social order, must remain the basis of civilisation for all those peoples that claim to be civilised.

The English edition of the present volume has received wide endorsement from both lay and medical press. Some of the press comments follow:

"The structure and function of the reproductive organs are clearly set out . . . the sections upon the problems of puberty and the sexual impulse are quite sane in their teaching. Facts that are disagreeable, some of which were till recently not accepted as facts, are faced, and the reasons for the conclusions upon debatable points are given."—*The Lancet* (*London*).

"This is a scientific treatise on the subject, dealing with the structure and function of the genital organs, menstruation, reproduction, pregnancy and its diagnosis, the sexual impulse, and impotence, as well as sterility, heredity and other kindred topics. It is a book which strikes the happy mean between too much and too little. It gives just those facts which are essential to a correct understanding of sex. The book is one which gives a very accurate and scientific account of the subject, and has the added advantage of being illustrated."—*The Medical Times* (*London*).

"The work has been written by two distinguished specialists, and is notable for its sane and practical viewpoint . . . There are preliminary chapters dealing with the physiology and anatomy of the male and female reproductive organs, reproduction and puberty. These are followed by chapters which throw into contrast the sexual impulse in man with that of woman . . . This book . . . will please those who wish to supplement their knowledge by the knowledge of scientific specialists."—*Health and Empire* (*Journal of the British Social Hygiene Council*).

" . . . Offers the sanest and most practical views of sexology and sexual hygiene that can be found . . . A clear conception of the anatomy and physiology, the structure and functions, of the male and female reproductive organs can be obtained from the preliminary chapters . . . The portion devoted to the sexual impulse in male is one that should be read and re-read by every father and son . . . no *saner* or simpler source book is to be found anywhere."—*The Gilmorehill Globe* (*Glasgow University, Glasgow*).

"It is a sane and practical account of the physical side of sex. —*The Prescriber* (*Edinburgh*).

"Drs. Buschke and Jacobsohn have collaborated upon a work which is frank, fearless and sensible. The whole problem of the sex instinct as it crops up in the daily life of the average individual is surveyed concisely and sagaciously. The authors' chief object has obviously been to furnish a safe and intelligent guide on the subject chosen. The book constitutes an eminently sane and practical account of the physical phase of sex as a basis on which to solve the difficulties of modern marriage."—*Montreal Daily Star.*

" . . . Gives a lucid account of the anatomy, physiology and hygiene of sex."—*The New Generation* (*London*).

"This excellently produced and well illustrated book, written by two doctors, is one of the most sensible which has ever been written on the subject. There are chapters upon abnormalities, eugenics, monogamy, heredity and venereal diseases, as well as the more strictly mechanical chapters."—*The Madras Mail* (*India*).

" . . . Will prove of value to those requiring information on the various aspects of sexual life."—*North-China Daily News.*

Bei Fragen zur Produktsicherheit wenden Sie sich bitte an:
If you have any questions regarding product safety,
please contact:

Walter de Gruyter GmbH
Genthiner Straße 13
10785 Berlin
productsafety@degruyterbrill.com